FATMAN
in
Recovery

FATMAN
in
Recovery

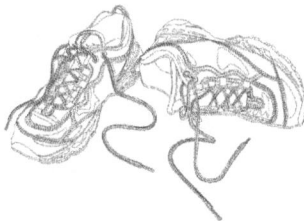

Tales from the Brink
of Obesity

AVVENTURA
PRESS

Cover and interior design by Lee Sebastiani & Lori Sebastiani,
Avventura Press
Cover photo: Leslie Bacinelli
Photos: Jay Sochoka

ISBN-13: 978-0-9761553-9-3

Published by
Avventura Press
133 Handley St.
Eynon PA 18403-1305
570-876-5817
www.avventurapress.com

1st printing October 2010
Printed in the United States of America

FOREWORD

When I met Jay Sochoka, he was running for his life.

A self-described "fat man in recovery," he once tipped the scales at more 300 pounds and had whittled himself down to a trim 198. He was about to run his fifth Steamtown Marathon, and was hoping to finish with a time that would qualify him for the Boston Marathon.

He had missed the mark by a mere 40 seconds the year before, greeted by his cheering family, including his father, Joe, who was dying and would not live to see his son run again. Jay carried his father's memory with him in the next race, and crossed the finish line convinced a higher power had nudged him forward when he needed it most.

Jay went on to run the Boston Marathon, and to do many other things the depressed, 300-pound, pack-a-day smoker he once was never had the energy or the ambition to dream, let alone achieve. "Anyone has the power within to do what I did," Jay told me that first time we met, and many times since. The way he sees it, life is a race between hope and fear, and victory depends on which the runner chooses to embrace.

"The process is a marathon, not a sprint," Jay says, and he means it.

One of the best parts of my job as a community journalist is meeting ordinary people who do extraordinary things. Their stories are inspiring, entertaining, and, most importantly, real. Stories don't come much better than Jay's, and I'm honored that he invited me to help him tell it.

Jay Sochoka is still running for his life. After finishing this book, don't be surprised if you find yourself running for yours, too.

—*Chris Kelly, July 17, 2010*

ACKNOWLEDGEMENTS

First of all, I would like to thank the three people who made my life possible. They are The Father, The Son, and The Holy Spirit. Without them I am nothing. Next, I would like to thank Mom and Dad. We have been down a long road, and it may have been bumpy in spots but I wouldn't trade you for the Bradys, The Cleavers, or all the tea in China. To my beloved wife and child: you complete my life. I also want to thank the rest of my family for always being there for me. To those of you I have shared the apple with (you'll find out what that means)— I can never repay all you have given to me. Then, there are the friends, and I mean the true friends, I have made in my life: Glenn Vignola, Jack Smedley, Frank Krantz IV, Bob Gilmartin, Jim Beers, Art Aubert, and Joey Marino. You are more than friends; you are family, and I am blessed to have met and gotten to know you. I can't thank Chris Kelly enough for believing in this book and taking the time to edit it. I'm truly honored that such a talented writer believes in what I wrote. A huge thanks to Avventura Press for taking a chance on someone whose biggest work before this was a 15-page history report on The Beatles in my freshman year of high school. Finally, I would like to thank you, the reader, for buying this book. I hope you enjoy reading it as much as I have enjoyed writing it.

Peace.

PREFACE

Everybody has a story.

Only a few people will actually tell it.

Hello and thank you for taking the time to take a peek into my life. Every word of this book is the God's honest truth. It may sound like a novel in spots but I swear to you this is nonfiction. The quotes are reproduced to the best of my "I partied my way through college" memory.

I hope this book makes you laugh and even makes you cry. It okay to cry you know. I hope it makes you say, "I've been there," or "He was in a tough spot and got out of it. So can I." I hope you realize that you can come up against seemingly insurmountable odds yet achieve the highest levels of personal success, because you can. It seems like there is no way that all of this could have happened to me, but I assure you it did. As unbelievable as this story sounds, it ALL happened.

Finally, I hope you come to a point, or are at a point, in your life, where you are as blessed as I have been. Just remember that "Through Him all things are possible."

God bless.

*The story of a fat kid
who grew up to be a fat man
who grew up to be me*

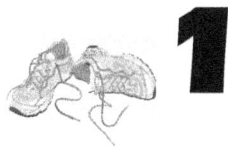

Redheaded Fat Kid

Oh please pick me. I don't want to be the last pick again.
I'm really not that bad a kickball player. C'mon—JUST
PICK ME!

I F I close my eyes, I can still see the playground at
Walter M. Schirra, Jr. Elementary School in Old Bridge,
New Jersey. I can still smell the turning leaves, feel
the cool slap of the autumn wind on the back of my sweat-
soaked neck and the thick churn in my gut as I stood on
line to be picked for kickball.

Every fat kid has a kickball story; most, more than one.
For fat kids, kickball is both a sport and a metaphor for
life. You are too slow and short-winded to be much use to
the team, and you take as many kicks as the ball. You are
expected to perform pathetically, and invariably do. In fact,
you're branded a loser before the game even begins.

In kickball as in life, captains do the picking. I can't
recall ever being a captain. I was only the first pick once
in my life and that was not until sixth grade. The kid who
picked me was fatter than I was.

I have many kickball stories, but they can all be rolled
into a single chilly fall afternoon from second grade. The

teams were all but set, just two people left on the block. It was down to me and a girl. A girl. Knowing how seriously my male peers took the risk of "cooties" infestation, I sauntered toward Anthony's team as confidently as any fat redhead can.

"Tara!" Anthony shouted, picking the girl over me.

I can still hear the laughter. Take the reaction Charlie Brown received when he delivered his forlorn Christmas tree and amplify it a thousand times a thousand. All these years later, it's as loud as ever. Crushed, I skulked over to the other team and took my place at the back of the line. It was where I belonged, and if I ever forgot it, there was always someone there to remind me.

To tell the truth, Tara was probably a better kickball player than me. I was far from athletic. When I played soccer, I was the kid who always finished laps last. There was one kid who routinely finished behind me, but he was "special." I asked my Dad why I couldn't be as good as Joey, the star of our team.

"Joey is just a natural born athlete," he said matter-of-factly. He didn't say, "And you are not," but I heard it just the same. It was the truth, and it hurt.

I was a classic late starter. I was about 18 months old when I started to walk. Mom was so worried she took me to a pediatric neurologist. She was convinced something was wrong with me. There wasn't. I was just slow getting out of the blocks. It would be a long time before I would hit my stride.

On top of being slow-starting, I was different. For years, I was the only redhead in the school. Add freckles and a few extra pounds and I may as well have had a "kick me" sign for a birthmark. Kids called me fat, fatty, fatso, chubby, husky, tub of lard, porker, and that was just elementary school. The language got more colorful — and more hurtful — as I got older.

Every Catholic fat kid with a kickball story also has a Buying My First Holy Communion Suit story. Mine was beige with a white shirt and white tie (Ah, those magical 70s). Up on the tailor's measuring stand, I was once again on uncomfortable display. I was a big kid, but I never felt so small.

"He's going to need a chubby," the tailor said. He just could not just keep his mouth shut and take us to where we needed to go. He had to say it. I wanted to hit him. To this day, I believe divine intervention kept me from doing it. Instead, I trudged to the husky section and picked out a suit.

The cause of my heaviness was no mystery. I was consuming more calories than I was burning. I ate too much. My whole family ate too much. My family is fond of saying we all starved to death in a previous life and are making up for it now. This is never truer than at Christmas. After three hours of hors d'oeuvres, we sit down to a four-course meal. After we open presents, it's time for dessert. Somehow, I always found room for all of it. Still do.

By some cruel twist of gastronomical fate, only Mom and I showed our love for eating. Dad could down anything and not gain an ounce. Once, he ate the entire dessert menu at a resort. Every fat person knows somebody like that. Believe me, it's tougher when he's your Dad.

I was born hungry. I was a week old when Mom started mixing rice cereal into my formula because I was "starving" in her eyes. Food will soothe a crying baby, and the remedy translates easily into childhood. Scraped knee? Have a cookie. Pain gone, crying stopped. Why go to the pharmacy when all the medicine you need is in the cookie jar?

There was a point in my early life when the Redheaded Fat Kid could have gone away for good. Dad drove by the high school, and I noticed that the football field was circled by a track. I was in kindergarten, so it was 1976, the year of the Montreal Olympics. Frank Shorter won the silver medal in the marathon, Steve Prefontaine had died in a car wreck before he could have another shot at Lasse Vieren in the 5K, and Bruce Jenner won the decathlon and got his picture on a Wheaties box. America was suddenly crazy about running.

At the time, no one was faster than "The Six Million Dollar Man," which, for obvious reasons was my favorite show. Steve Austin survived a brutal plane crash and was rebuilt from head to toe. Using bionics, doctors had made him, "better...stronger...faster." I can still hear the theme music behind the monologue. Steve Austin could jump over fences, lift cars and see things from a mile away. He even fought Bigfoot once. He was my hero, and I had the running suit to prove it.

Seeing the track and the thin, fast people sprinting around it, I decided that I wanted to put my jogging suit to good use.

"Dad, I want to run."

"OK, son, we'll go to the track on Sunday after church."

Mass could not end soon enough that day. I was bouncing in my pew just itching to go to the track and run. There were other people running when we pulled up, and in my Six Million Dollar Man running suit I took off. I just wanted to get around the track once without having to walk. I got around and Dad asked, "How do you feel?"

"Fine," I said.

"Good. Run another one."

I went around again and no worse for wear was sent for a third lap. After three, I still felt fine and went for a fourth lap. I wanted to keep going, but Dad told me I had just run a mile and should stop. I was hooked.

Sunday became track day. I ran a one-mile track meet every week. I remember running with an old man named Ray. I remember his name because it rhymed with mine. I can still see him in his blue T-shirt and white sweat band around his head. He would run alongside me and give me tips. On one particularly windy day, he told me to lean forward and dip my head down when running into a strong wind. This adjustment allows the wind to slip over you a little easier than just standing tall. I still use that trick.

Running also taught me the "Thrill of victory and the agony of defeat." I'll never forget my PR (Personal Record) time from back then—12 minutes and 13 seconds. I actually finished ahead of a handful of adults that day. It was a great feeling, an "I didn't win the race, but won anyway," moment. Coach, I don't know his name I just knew him as "Coach", told my parents that I should sign up for a cross country race the following week.

It was one of those days that can define your life, for better or worse. We got to the park, were given a walking tour of the course, and got on the starting line. The gun went off and I was instantly left in everyone's dust.

The first part of the course looped back around to the starting line where the crowd was gathered. I was running at full tilt and I couldn't even see another runner on the course. "Turn on the gas!" someone yelled. I tried, I really did, but I could not go any faster.

With tears streaming down my face I stopped and broke down crying. I remember Mom gently leading me off the course. I officially recorded my first DNF (Did Not Finish) at the age of 5.

Looking back, it's clear what went wrong. I did not run my own race. Had I just settled down, ignored the guy telling me to step on it, and ran at my own pace, I would have finished with no problem. Instead, I ran like I had a chance at beating 50 or so adults. I guess at age five it's hard to see the big picture. I left defeated that day, but it did not turn me off from running.

My pediatrician took care of that. When Mom told him what I had been doing on the track, he had two words: "Absolutely not!" In his opinion, running on a track was much too risky for my young joints. My running career was over at age five. For some reason, playing tag (running for your life) for an hour was fine. Playing soccer (running with a ball) was OK too, but running around a track was simply verboten.

Today, pediatricians would kill to see a kid so passionate about running. In our super-sized society, I would have been encouraged to keep going. Instead, I was diagnosed with an unhealthy appetite for exercise and practically ordered to be more sedentary. The Redheaded Fat Kid was on his way to the back of the kickball line, where he would languish for—years.

It was where I belonged, and if I ever forgot it, there was always someone there to remind me.

2

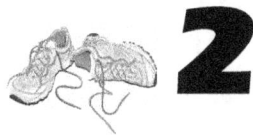

If Every Day Were Kindergarten, I Would Have Stayed in School

WAS there anything better than kindergarten? It is our introduction to the concept of the workday, but somehow learning shapes, basic math and how to spell and write didn't seem like work. Maybe it was because our minds were so pliable back then that we could suck it all up without too much effort. It felt like play time.

And after play time came snack time, which is our introduction to associating eating with recreation. I can still taste the Twinkies and milk. I'll bet you can, too.

Kindergarten is a judgment-free zone. There is no color barrier, no intelligence barrier and no shape barrier. We were all just a bunch of kids having the time of our young lives. We came in different sizes, shapes, and colors and had different levels of potential, but those differences were taken in stride, if they were noticed at all.

Maybe the best thing about kindergarten was the brevity of hours—in by nine, out by eleven-thirty. Who wouldn't love a work week like that? My class had a jobs list. Each week, you were assigned a different task. They were all fun, but three stick out in my memory:

Flag Holder: You got to hold the flag during the Pledge of Allegiance. With great power comes great responsibility, and holding the flag commanded a lot of respect.

Milk Stand: Everyone wanted milk, and you were the guy who could make it happen. Customers would line up neatly and you would dispense the heavenly nectar. If someone got rowdy, you had the power to send him or her to the back of the line. It's a lot of authority in the hands of a Twinkie-fueled five-year-old.

Line Leader: This was akin to the presidency. You got to lead the class to the gym and anywhere else it had to go. Even the teacher walked alongside the line. It was a great honor to lead the brigade, even if you never got to choose the direction.

In a society obsessed with getting ahead, kindergarten is one of the last times it is acceptable to talk about the pure joy of learning. If there were grades handed out in kindergarten, I don't remember them. I understand that grades are necessary, and that periodic evaluations of skills and aptitudes are essential to building a strong society. I won't argue any of that. It occurs to me, though, that if schooling after kindergarten were more focused on the joy of learning than the struggle to achieve, we might build a happier, healthier society. Grades are meant to be measurements, not the yardstick itself, which brings me to the only bad thing about kindergarten:

It's over before you know it.

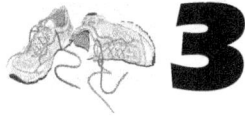

3

Meet the Parents

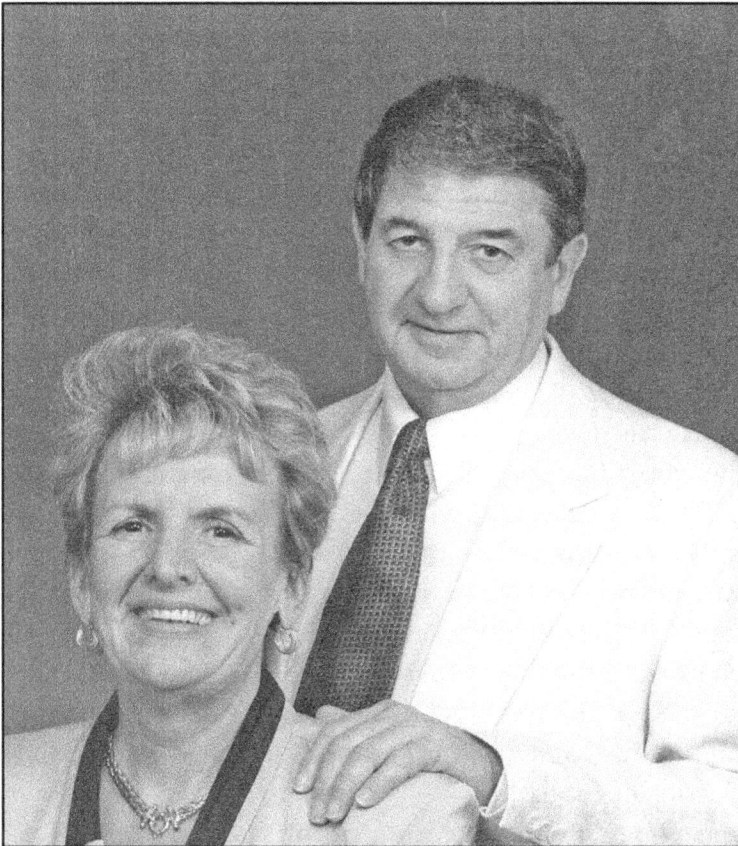

Judy and Joe Sochoka
30th anniversary, 1998

I AM very fortunate to have been raised by my folks. We were not the Rockefellers, but there wasn't much I ever wanted for. Any toy I wanted as a kid—Santa brought it. If he didn't, I'd get it for my birthday, for a good grade, or even for no good reason other than Mom and Dad wanted me to have it.

I am an only child, which is the leading cause of spoiled brats. I took offense to the characterization as a child, but as an adult with a boy of my own, I am on the paying end of the arrangement, financially and emotionally. Besides the toys, I got to play hockey, soccer, and baseball, although I was never much good at any of them. As most spoiled brats do, I became accustomed to a certain standard of living and did not know or care how much my parents sacrificed to provide for me. As a parent firmly anchored in the middle class and sometimes struggling to keep my family afloat, I now understand how much my parents gave up to make me happy, and it is a debt I can never repay.

Joseph John Sochoka was born on September 4, 1937, in Scranton, Pennsylvania. He was the son of Joseph and Mary Sochovka (the 'V' was somehow omitted on Dad's birth certificate). He had a brother, John, and a sister, Mary Ann. He graduated from Scranton Technical High School in 1955 and went into the Air Force soon after. I can't tell you what it was like for him to grow up in the Sochovka family homestead, because he didn't talk about it much. He told me he played baseball and basketball and palled around with friends, but he only rarely talked about growing up in his home on Dorothy Street in the Tripp Park section of Scranton.

When he did, it was not a happy story.

"It was a nightmare," Dad once told me of his childhood. That is all he ever told me.

Judith Ellen Prosnak was born on November 16, 1942, also in Scranton. She has a sister named Evelyn. I called her parents Paul and Josephine "Mama" and "Pop" and could not have been more blessed to have them as grandparents. Mama and Pop were good parents, too. They didn't have a lot of money, but their children never felt poor. Mom also recalls that her parents never had a fight in front of the kids. This gave Mom an unrealistically idyllic view of marriage.

Mom holds the considerable distinction of being the first college graduate in the family. She graduated from Marywood College (now Marywood University) in 1964. At the time, it was a Catholic college for young women. Mom was taught by nuns all her life as she went to Holy Rosary elementary and high schools. Needless to say, Marywood didn't host many campus keg parties. Smoking a cigarette was about as risqué as it got. Mom got her degrees in special and elementary education and took a teaching job at John F. Kennedy Elementary School in Jamesburg, New Jersey.

My parents met at a bar called O'Toole and Andre's in Scranton. Dad's famous pickup line, "Haven't I met you before?" actually worked. Mom wasn't all that interested at first. She lied about where she lived in New Jersey, but as fate would have it, Dad happened to be living in the next town over at the time.

Mom and Dad were married on June 12, 1968. They moved to Old Bridge, New Jersey, where she taught school and he worked for American Airlines. Photo albums suggest they had a good time before I came into the picture. They traveled for free because of Dad's job, and when they were home they threw parties with the neighbors.

On August 10, 1971, I came into the picture, just ahead of the train wreck. Dad walked away from his job at American to try his luck in a pyramid scheme. This left us without health insurance and Mom as our sole source of income. She needed to get back on her feet as soon as possible.

There was a time when you could not leave the hospital after having a baby without dropping another package out the back door. Mom faked a bowel movement, and when the nurse came in to see it, Mom said she had accidentally flushed it. The nurse believed her, and we went home to 24 Island Drive as a family. She did this on a Saturday, because she knew the billing office would be closed. Dad said it was all he could do to drive the car. He looked back at me every chance he had.

The story always made Dad laugh, but good humor soon became rare in the Sochoka household. Dad battled violent mood swings and was eventually diagnosed with Manic Depression (known today as the trendier Bipolar Disorder). Alcoholism and bipolar disorder are a more volatile mix than flame and gasoline. When Dad was feeling good, life was great. When Dad was down, he took us with him. Days would pass without him uttering a word, always followed by fits of rage that invariably concluded with a tearful apology. Looking back, it was like clockwork.

Mom and I were ridiculously codependent. We planned our lives around Dad's moods, which is no way to live. My stomach would fill with knots as the inevitable storm brewed. You knew it was coming, and there was nothing you could do to stop it. Dad's childhood home life ended up being a template for mine. It really was a nightmare. Somehow my parents stayed married. Divorce, after all, is not in the Catholic vocabulary.

In fairness, there were far more good times than bad. Dad came light years farther in battling his demons. I would not trade my parents for the Bradys or the Cleavers. Every childhood has its rough spots, and mine helped make me who I am.

I only remember Dad hitting me once. I went after someone with a wiffle ball bat and Dad caught me doing it. He slapped me on the small of the back. I can still feel the sting. He vowed that day that he would never lay another hand on me, and he kept his word.

Dad eventually managed to quit drinking. I don't recall him going to meetings, he just stopped. While he did not drink, he was bitterly resentful of those who did. It's called being a dry drunk. Dry drunks can be just as unpleasant as active alcoholics, something Mom and I would learn the hard way.

Without the "self-medication" the alcohol provided, Dad had no buffer between him and his demons. This was long before psychotherapy and counseling became common. Back then, mental illness was highly stigmatizing. You were either crazy or you weren't. Going to a therapist was admitting defeat. It was for the mentally weak, and Dad would have none of it.

Instead, Dad shared his personal nightmare with Mom and me, and we just kept praying for the day when we all would wake up.

"I came into the picture...."

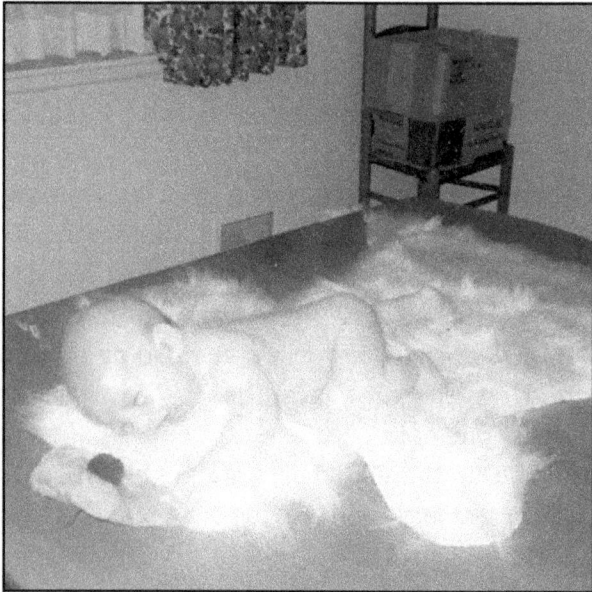

Bare-arsed on bearskin, 1971

4

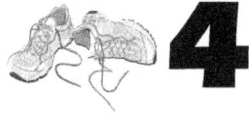

My First Diet and the Aftermath

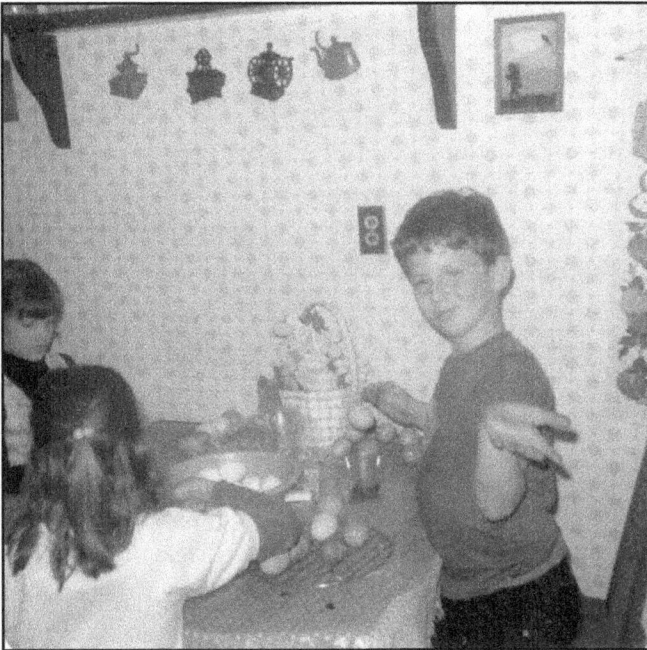

Dad used this third grade photo
to show me how thin I wasn't

OM was just coming off of her most successful weight loss episode ever. She wanted to be a certain size for my First Communion pictures and had pulled it off. Years later, she told me she was so thin, she could see the bones in her back.

The weight was starting to creep back on and she was dieting again. The refrigerator door was papered with meal plans. I was in third grade, and my excess weight made me a favorite target of classmates. Mom knew I was hurting and my weight was the cause. She suggested I diet with her. I was reluctant, but I desperately wanted the teasing to stop. Soon enough, my food list was tacked up on the fridge next to Mom's and I became friends with the food scale, weighing and measuring everything that went into my mouth. The same scale is in Mom's kitchen to this day.

The restrictiveness of the food plan was barbaric by today's standards. Chicken or fish. Red meat, pork, and other meats were out. This was long before pork became the other white meat. I ate a lot of chicken with the skin peeled off, which without breading and seasoning is the epicurean equivalent of a Wednesday in February—gray, gloomy and endless. To this day, I rarely eat baked chicken.

Breakfast was a single scrambled egg with Pam cooking spray. No butter. If we had toast, it was dry. Butter and jelly? A fantasy. Skim milk over a cup of bland cereal was as sexy as it got. Gone were pancakes, waffles, and my all-time favorite, French toast. Eating for enjoyment was a thing of the past. This was eating for mere existence.

In one of those brutal ironies that are so much a part of school life, the lunches that were intended to slim me down and end the taunting made me stick out even more. While my classmates lined up for school lunches, I ate alone. I was usually finished by the time my friends got back to the table with their pizza, cheeseburgers, and other high-fat delights. My fare was chicken roll on thin bread with a piece of fruit. Chicken roll is not all that healthy, but the portions were so small that the caloric content was almost irrelevant. I got an ounce of meat on the sandwich if I was lucky. On special days, Mom packed me a fruit roll-up instead of a piece of fruit. It was like winning the lunchroom lottery.

I'm convinced I was the only third grader drinking diet soda. This was before Nutrasweet, Splenda and other modern sweeteners, and before saccharin was determined to "cause cancer in laboratory animals" and a general sense of despair among sugar-deprived third-graders. There was no Diet Coke or Diet Pepsi. The market belonged to Tab, Fresca, and Diet Dr. Pepper. The latter was my favorite once I got used to it. Like anything God-awful, if you ingest enough of it, you can almost enjoy it. Juicy Juice, the 100 percent fruit juice, and water were the other beverages I was allowed.

They came in handy when washing down salad. Salad was as much a coping mechanism as a source of nutrition. Load up on salad, chase it with water, and you can feel full after even the skimpiest meal. There was sparse use of dressing because of the ridiculous fat content. I don't think light dressing or light mayonnaise existed at the time. A monster salad is still a staple in my eating routine. It helps give me that, "I just ate a whole cow" feeling at dinner with out any of the guilt. Go easy on the dressing and you can't go wrong. You fill up on a natural product that is essentially water and fiber, which go out as fast as they come in. A word to the wise: don't stray too far from a restroom until your body adjusts to the mass fiber influx. The first seven days can be a gastrointestinal adventure.

My third-grade eating plan afforded me so many ounces of protein, starches, fats, and fruits. There were not only restrictions on quantity, but on the types of food in each category. For example, peas, corn and potatoes were not considered vegetables, but starches, and were heavily restricted. Of course, peas and corn were the only two vegetables I had a taste for at the time.

I starved the first week. No matter how much I begged, Mom held the line. It got easier in week two, but I still felt like inmates at the state prison were eating better than me. It was like being sentenced to food jail, and Mom was the no-nonsense warden. Parole was out of the question.

And then a funny thing happened. I lost weight. I was thin. When I started playing little league baseball, I was at my heaviest. At the end of the season, I couldn't find myself in the opening day picture. I had changed so much in those two months, I didn't recognize myself. I had won the battle of the bulge, but had no idea the war was only beginning.

The main reason the diet worked was bribery. For every five pounds I lost, Mom bought me a new "Star Wars" action figure. I amassed quite a collection over those few months. The grand prize for reaching my goal weight was designer jeans. Any new fourth-grader who expected to climb socially knew well the names Jordache, Sasoon, Sergio Valenti, and Brittania. I remember going into Abraham & Strauss (a.k.a. A&S) in the Woodbridge Mall, which was the biggest on the east coast at the time, to pick out the jeans. I came home with Sergios and Brittanias. I don't remember the measurements, but my waist either equaled or was less than my inseam. They didn't make designer genes for plus-sized people. Victory was mine, and it had bright gold stitches across its tight, blue butt.

I was so excited to wear my new jeans that I could not wait for the first day of school, quite a change from the usual feeling of dread that usually started about two weeks before going back. I put on a pair of Sergios Valentes and strutted to school. At the playground, my "friends" let me in on a crushing bit of news: designer jeans were so last year. Levi's were the new rage.

Today, I am a card-carrying metrosexual. I wear Express jeans, carry a man purse, get my hands manicured, and I don't care who knows it. In fourth grade, I lacked self confidence and was hypersensitive to being teased. The ribbing I took over the designer jeans was just as bad as the abuse I took for being fat. Heavy or thin, I just could not win.

Soon after, the dieting stopped. I remember pigging out on an Easter basket that spring and it all going downhill from there. By the next school year, the red-headed fat kid was back, this time in a pair of loose-fit Levi's.

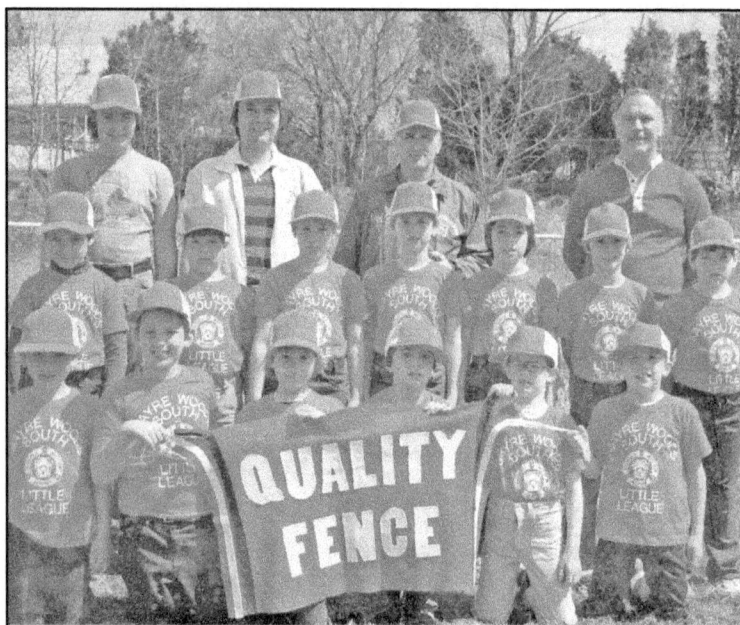

*The baseball photo I couldn't recognize myself in
(I'm holding the far left side of the banner)*

5

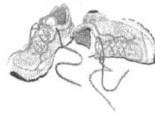

Off The Wagon...
And Getting Back On

It started with one free drink and nearly ended in a divorce.

Dad liked to go down to Atlantic City to play the slots. The casinos push free drinks to loosen up gamblers' inhibitions and wallets. The average sucker usually walks away a few bucks lighter but none the worse for wear, but for compulsive gamblers and alcoholics, the stakes are astronomically higher.

Dad couldn't say no to anything free. He took the drink. He probably felt that he could have just one and walk away, which would be like me just eating one Oreo cookie. Before I know it, I'm through the whole bag.

Starting out, Dad drank occasionally, having one or two drinks and feeling like he was in control. Soon, he was drinking a few times a week, the quantities were increasing and his control was slipping. Before he realized it, he was back in the trouble he had been in five years earlier.

It all came to a head in December of my fourth grade year. It still puts my stomach in knots just to think about it, but I have to tell you this story to tell you another one.

We were decorating the Christmas tree. Mom was there, along with my cousins Michele and Paul, as they always were, to decorate the tree. Dad was not. He was never a fan of Christmas back then (it brought back bad childhood memories) and didn't do much when it came to putting ornaments on the tree. He would at least hang out in the living room and play Christmas records on a console system that looked like a bar with speakers. Lost in the Ray Coniff Singers' harmonies, I got caught up in the festivities and kind of forgot that Dad wasn't there.

Only after the tree was decorated and I was upstairs watching the "Dukes of Hazzard" did I stop to think about why Dad wasn't home. I asked Mom, but I don't remember getting an answer. She certainly did not say, "He's out getting plastered."

I don't remember much about the next week, except that it was very quiet. When it was quiet in my childhood home, that just meant a storm was brewing.

I slept through it. I didn't hear the shouting. I did not hear Dad leave Mom.

I woke up and Mom told me my Baba (Russian for grandmother) was sick and Dad had to go to Pennsylvania. The next thing I knew, Mama and Pop were down about three days earlier that they normally would have been for Christmas. Dad would always stay at Mama and Pop's when he went to Scranton. Something just did not add up. I kept asking questions, and Mom finally admitted what happened and under what circumstances.

The bottom line was that I didn't know if Dad was going to come back. Ever. I thought for sure that my parents were headed for a divorce. Having friends with divorced parents, I knew exactly what that meant, and I didn't like the idea at all.

It was Christmas Eve, and that meant it was time to go to my Aunt Evelyn (Mom's sister) and Uncle Mike's house for prayer, a feast, and of course, opening presents. It is the holiest night of the year, and it was an absolute requirement to be at that house on Christmas Eve. All these years later, it still is. No exceptions.

I had resigned myself to the fact that Dad was going to miss this one. Mom and I drove to Aunt's Evelyn's house and the festivities commenced with hors d'oeurvres. I started having fun with my cousins Paul and Michele, playing Christmas songs on the organ in the hallway. When I walked into the kitchen, Dad was suddenly there.

"Dad!" I shouted as I ran over to him and gave him a huge hug. "Where did you go?"

"I went to Pennsylvania," he said. "Baba was sick."

"No you didn't. I know what happened," was my answer, and the conversation stopped. I guess he figured that I was too smart for my own good, and, since he didn't want to make things worse, he kept his mouth shut.

Regardless of what happened, I was thrilled to see him. I wanted him to stay, even if it was just for the night.

"Can we keep him?" I asked Mom, as if Dad were a stray puppy. Looking back now, I probably wasn't that far off.

I don't remember getting an answer. The next thing I knew, I was being ushered into the basement by my cousin and Godfather Paul. When the coast was clear, I was given the green light to come upstairs. Dad was gone. Mom told him he couldn't stay. Dinner went on as planned.

A few days later, Dad showed up at home. I was happy to see him, but worried about the fight that was likely to happen. Somehow, it didn't. Dad was repentant. Dad, Mom, Mama, and Pop were discussing things in the bedroom. I popped my head in to see three people standing on the far side of the bed and Dad lying down on it crying. It was the first time I ever saw him cry. I didn't think he even knew how. My heart broke for him.

Mom was not so moved. She took me into the living room and sat me down. I knew what was coming. "I want a divorce," she said. I was furious. I didn't say a thing, but I remember what my young mind thought: "Why do you want to do this to us? Why do you want to break us up? WHY DO YOU WANT TO TAKE MY DADDY AWAY FROM ME?"

It never happened. My parents did not divorce. Dad was allowed to stay, but not without conditions. He had to go to rehab. He needed to quit drinking. He was gone the next day, but I knew he would be home, eventually.

Mom made life as normal as possible during the rest of the holiday break. She was a teacher, so we had the time off together. Dad was cut off from society so he could dry out. We wouldn't be able to visit him until New Year's Day, so we were on our own for New Year's Eve. We used to go to a Polynesian restaurant called The Islander in Matawan, N.J. We would drink virgin piña coladas and eat pu pu platter, as well as this dish called the Hawaii 5-0, which was pork, water chestnuts, and vegetables stir-fried in a white sauce and served with a side of pork-fried rice. It tasted as good as it sounds. Mom and I had a good time, but I remember hoping the two of us eating alone would not become a family tradition.

On New Year's Day, we were off to Perth Amboy General Hospital to visit Dad. I was very excited. I felt like it had been forever since I had seen him. We went into the reception room, which was about the size of a school cafeteria.

Apparently, Dad wasn't the only alcoholic or addict in the area. The room was packed with visitors. I remember seeing Dad come down the stairs. I jumped into his arms and kissed him. The whole visit was a blur, with the exception of a conversation we had.

"Do you know what I am?" Dad asked.

"You're kind of an alcoholic," I replied.

"No, son," he said. "I am an alcoholic, and I will always be an alcoholic."

I learned something that day. Once you were labeled an alcoholic, it stayed with you for life. The best you could do was become a recovering alcoholic. Dad went to Alcoholics Anonymous and got his 90 meetings in 90 days pin. After that, he went to meetings at least once a week. He had a sponsor. He was doing everything he could to stay in Mom's good graces. Things on the home front were good.

And then they changed again. Dad wound up going to a new treatment facility called Fair Oaks. I thought that he was drinking again. He wasn't. One morning, he went to Mom crying. He told her that he felt like he was going to kill himself. Mom stayed home from work that day. Thank God for that. I couldn't imagine what would have happened if she didn't.

Dad was diagnosed manic-depressive, and I believe he was put on lithium. I don't know the specifics, because this was the early 1980s. Mental illness was not talked about back then. It was far more stigmatizing then than it is today, and today it is still bad.

Psychotherapy was not an option. Dad saw needing a "shrink" as a weakness and would have nothing to do with it. He would be placed on lithium, go to AA, and we would hope for the best.

For the most part, it worked. Life went back to normal, or what passes for that in a classic dysfunctional and codependent household. The folks still fought, and it still killed me to hear it, but we never again had a time as hard as the Christmas after Dad took one free drink.

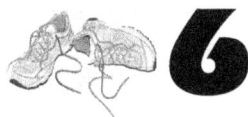

Flashes of Adolescence

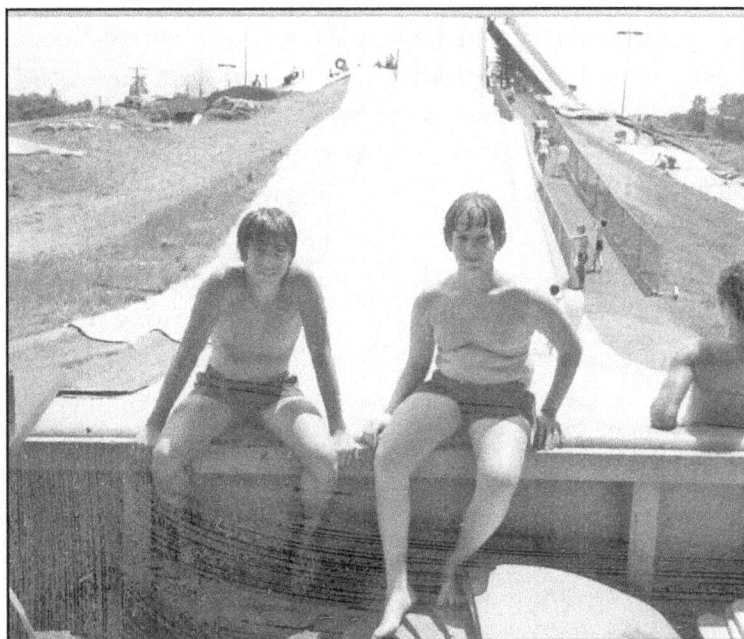

Teenage Buddha
(Glenn Vicaola is the skinny one)

A DOLESCENCE is like a race between your body and your mind.

Your body has a huge head start, and your mind is always running off in so many directions, it has almost no chance of catching up before serious damage has been done. Between 13 and 18, you are not an adult, but you are also no longer a child. If you ask me, you're still a kid until you're at least 21. (Unless, of course, you're a kid with a kid; then you grow up really fast.)

If I had a time machine, I would go back to my teens just to punch myself in the face. Back then, I thought I could kick anyone's ass, regardless of their age, but the truth is that I would have had my ass handed to me instead.

Dad taught me how to defend myself from an early age. I was instructed to never start a fight. I remember being about four years old and he would spar with me while kneeling. He wouldn't clobber me, but he would throw punches. When he was done with the session, he would always throw the fight by letting me land a combination of punches and "knock him out." Obviously, I was too small to do any real damage. This exercise was meant to teach me a few lessons.

Here are The Big Three:

Keep your guard up.

Don't lead with your head.

Don't telegraph your punches. Telegraphing, for the pugilistically challenged, means that you wind up your punch so much (think Popeye revving up before clocking Bluto) that your opponent can see it coming and blocks it. If you're not landing punches, you are not doing damage, and you are going to lose the fight.

I don't remember how old I was when Dad started to fight me standing up. As I got older, his punches got progressively harder and faster. This wasn't child abuse; it was learning self-defense. As I got older, I hit harder, too.

One day, our sparring session turned into a full-on fight. The punches were fast and furious, and I was feeling what Dad was throwing. I don't know what got into us that day but we were really at it. Our defenses were tight. Nothing serious was getting in.

Then Dad made a mistake.

He telegraphed a punch. I saw his right hook coming, and ducked it as I moved left. His whole right side was wide open. I came up and launched the most brutal uppercut I could muster. It was a direct hit. I could feel the power of the punch landing on his ribcage.

He dropped, waving his glove at me.

"No more," he wheezed. He stayed down for at least 10 seconds. Knockout. He had taught me well, and I learned my lessons. I asked him many times, but we didn't box again for at least a year.

When we did, it wasn't the same, and we soon traded our boxing gloves for wounding words, which can take the wind out of you just as surely as a well-placed uppercut.

We'll explore that later. Let's take a spin around the lake.

My family has a cottage at Newton Lake in Northeastern Pennsylvania, and I've had a boat since I was 13. I paid $3,000 of the $7,000 price, and Dad kicked in the rest.

Life at the lake was and is awesome. Spending my summers—especially in my teens— there was a blessing I for which I can never express enough thanks. Of course, I didn't always see it that way. Since I always had The Lake in my life, I took it for granted. It wasn't until I started working full-time that I realized how fortunate I was to have it.

There was a pack of teenagers up there and we all had boats. One day, we'd ski behind my boat, and behind someone else's the next. All of us were taught to drive boats from a very young age, and we knew just how far we could push the envelope. I don't recall anyone ever being seriously hurt.

We would ski all day and fish all night. All the angst and pressure and emotional conflicts of teendom melted into the waves like the evening sun. There's nothing wrong with the average teenager that can't be cured by watching the moon cross dark water. When I die, The Lake is what I expect Heaven to look like. It is a paradise on earth, and I owe it all to Dad, who worked hard to give it to me.

Many times alone on the water, I have reflected on the times Dad and I fought. The memories are painful, but The Lake has a way of soothing the deepest hurts. After all, God made The Lake, and he made me and Dad, too. It helps to remember that, and for some reason, being in a boat makes that easier.

I was 15 when Dad and I had what I recall as our worst fight. It was a February morning and it was snowing hard. He said something deeply hurtful to Mom that I will not repeat here. He always did go for the throat in a fight.

It went bad fast. Divorce came up. Mom told him to get out. Then it got truly ugly. Be warned: This next part contains some R-rated language. I'm sorry about that, but if I want you to understand where I'm coming from, I've got to keep it real.

The words were out of my mouth before I knew they were coming.

"Fuck you!" I screamed at Dad.

He was clearly stunned. It took him a few seconds to respond, but when he did, he held nothing back.

"Fuck me?" he raged. "Fuck you! My father would have put me through a fucking wall if I said that to him!"

He was right. There was no way Dad would have gotten away with saying that to Joe Sr. I was looking for a fight. I was hoping he would throw a punch at me. I was ready to hit him back. I knocked him out once, and knew I could do it again. I think that was the reason he didn't hit me. He was afraid of the outcome. Physically, I had the advantage. Verbally, he had an ace in the hole.

"I have news for you," he spat out in a venomous tone. "I was married before."

I was stunned. Crushed. Speechless. I started crying. What he said hurt. The way he said it hit harder than any punch. He had knocked me down, but not out. Consumed with rage, I got about three inches from his face and screamed the three words no parent wants to hear from a child: "I HATE YOU!"

Instantly, the fight stopped. He didn't have a comeback for that one. It felt good to hurt him. Only after having a son years later did I understand how painful it must have been for him. If Dad loved me a tenth as much as I love my child, it must have crushed him to hear me say those words.

Dad went upstairs to pack his things to leave. I began to feel awful. Mom asked me to go upstairs and talk him out of going. It was a very codependent request, but I probably would have gone on my own.

When I got to the top of the stairs, Dad had his back turned to me as he packed his bag. He was crying.

"My God," I thought. "What have I done?"

I asked him not to go, and he didn't say a word. He just turned around and we embraced. We both sobbed uncontrollably. We had our fights after that, especially as my teen years played out, but none ever came close to that day.

Most importantly, I never said those three words to my father again.

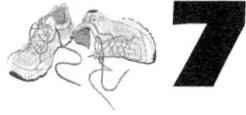

The One

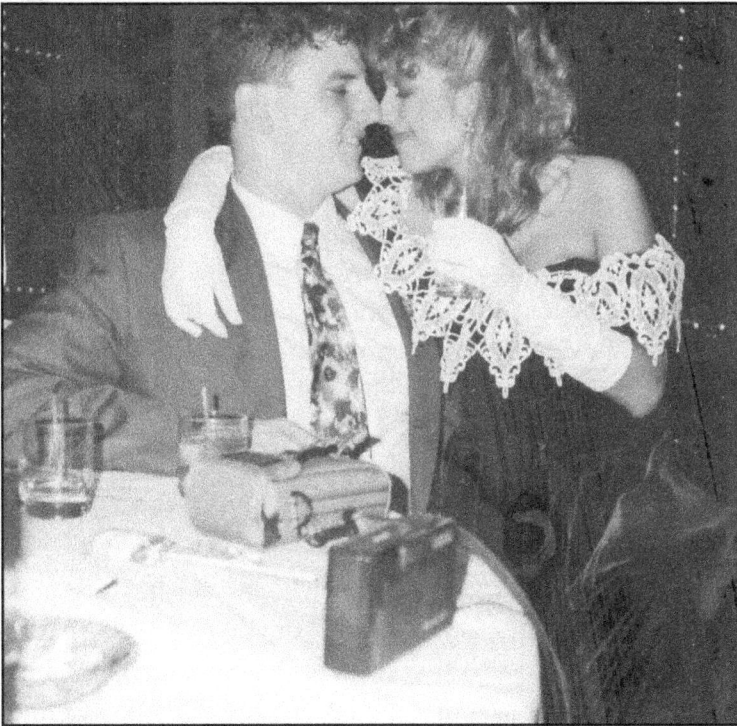

Jay and Sheryl Lynn

I AM convinced that nothing happens by coincidence. Do I believe there is a God? Absolutely. How do I know this? A priest told me so. Just kidding. My interactions with God are on a much more personal level. I've had some one on one time with Him, and we will talk about a few of those moments later. This moment is about how I met The One. The woman who would become my wife: Sheryl Lynn.

Ever notice how you find something when you are not looking for it? It's like when you find your spare set of keys after you have given up looking for them. That pretty much describes how I met Sheryl. I wasn't looking for a girlfriend. I had three acquaintances that I saw on a rotating basis. I had just been dumped out of a serious relationship, and I in no way wanted to get serious again. I was planning to go back to my last year at Philadelphia College of Pharmacy and Science a very eligible bachelor.

I was working a stand at the Dunmore Street Festival (in Dunmore, PA) selling T-shirts when she showed up.

It was August 13, 1993, and we were selling these shirts that had Warner Bros. characters dressed in NFL uniforms. I was firmly rooted in Eagles and Cowboys country, and those shirts were selling fast. "Do you have any more Dallas shirts in an Extra Large?" a voice asked.

I looked up, and this time I noticed her. This absolutely adorable young woman. She was quietly beautiful—not all tramped out like some women who know they are good looking dress. She was wearing a T-shirt, a pair of shorts, and wore glasses, but there was something very striking about her. She had the face of a model and the body to match. It might have taken me a few extra seconds to answer her.

"No, I don't, but I'll have more tomorrow. I'll put one aside," I said, trying to seal the deal in more ways than one.

"That would be great," she said, "but I have a family reunion, so I'll be here later."

"No problem. It will be waiting for you," I promised.

The conversation did not end there. We talked for at least an hour, as I tried to work at the same time. The boss was getting a little ticked because I wasn't working hard enough. He said people were waving money in front of me, and I wasn't seeing them. He was probably right. I definitely had tunnel vision that night. She left, and I was already looking forward to seeing her again.

The next day we got a new shipment of shirts and I immediately grabbed an XL Dallas Cowboys shirt, put it in a plastic bag, and stapled a piece of paper with the words, "DO NOT SELL" on it. It was a good thing I did. She wasn't there yet, and we sold all of the Cowboys shirts we had.

I was giving somebody his change when a voice rang out, "You creep! You didn't save me a shirt!"

She was wearing contact lenses, so it took me an extra second or two to find her. When I did I reached under the table and pulled out the hermetically sealed bag. I had a Cheshire Cat grin on my face. She smiled back. I sold her the shirt, and she didn't go anywhere. We started talking again.

We talked about everything. She loved *Phantom of the Opera*. I was a huge fan of the play. She said that nobody ever beat her at Trivial Pursuit, and I replied that I had the same problem. I even challenged her to a game. I asked her what bars she liked to go to and she said that she rarely went out to them. "What are you, anti-social?" I asked and almost overplayed my hand. Thankfully, she wasn't offended. She told me she would rather a quiet night at home.

She stayed so long that I met her Mom Frani and Dad Dave. Dave even tried to negotiate a better deal on an Eagles shirt. I got him to pay bust out retail for it. It's all about supply and demand. I met the folks already and we seemed to hit it off okay. That is always a hurdle to try and clear.

The festival was coming to a close, and she would be gone soon. I had my phone number already written on a card. "I won't call you," she said, "but here's my number." She gave me a piece of paper with her number and a smiley face on it. That was a good sign. Later she told me that she would use a star and smiley face and a heart to symbolize "Faith, Hope, and Love" respectively. She was hoping I would call.

"I'll call you Monday at nine o'clock." It was about the time I got home from my other job tending bar.

"Okay."

Monday Night, 9:01 p.m.

She answered the phone. She sounded really happy. We immediately started talking and talking and talking. During the conversation, I made the mental note that she liked pizza with pepperoni and black olives. That would come in handy in the future.

I asked if I could see her, and she said yes. I would see her that Wednesday at 9 p.m. I don't know how I managed to sleep that night or the next. I was that excited.

Wednesday, August 18, 1993.

I finished wiping down the bar and high-tailed it to Dunmore. I was low on gas, but I figured that into the plan. I would go to Grande Pizza (one of her favorites) order a large pie with pepperoni and black olives then go and fill up my tank. I got to the place and ordered the pie.

I ran back to my car, and it would not start. I was out of gas. Luckily enough, there was a gas station about two blocks away. I huffed and puffed my way to the gas station

(I was still a heavyset, run-only-when-chased kind of guy) and bought a gallon of gas. I ran back to my car and put it in.

I checked my watch and it was 9:05. I was already late. I ran to a pay phone and called her. No answer. She was waiting for me in front of her apartment. She couldn't hear the phone ring. I picked up the pizza, started the car, and went back to the gas station and topped off my tank. I then drove like a maniac to get to Sheryl's apartment. I swear that there were no less than 90 stop signs from the pizza parlor to her apartment. I was a good 15 minutes late.

She was in front of her apartment as she said she would be. I honked to her and parked the car.

"I ran out of gas," I said. "I tried to call. I'm sorry. Smell the gas on my hand if you don't believe me."

She believed me. We went upstairs and ate pizza while I schooled her at Trivial Pursuit. I wouldn't throw a game for anybody. Not even for someone I wanted to see more often. She lost gracefully. After the game we talked some more.

She showed me around her apartment. We sat down, and I told her how good I was at giving shoulder rubs. While I was rubbing her shoulders, she stopped talking and turned her face toward me. I ducked away. I then realized that she wanted to kiss me. The next time she turned her head our lips locked.

Three hours later, we were still kissing. It was beyond romantic. All I wanted to do was kiss her. She kissed me all the way to my car. I was already in love with her.

Sheryl was not moving quite as fast I was. She wasn't looking for a boyfriend, because she just had her heart broken in a relationship. Neither of us was looking, but we found each other. It was meant to be.

I introduced Sheryl to my parents, and they took an immediate liking to her. This sparked a very interesting conversation in our blossoming relationship. "Your Dad told me you have other girlfriends." I was speechless. I have no idea why he said this. It may have been true until August 18, 1993, at 9:15 p.m. My casual dating days were over and I told her so.

We were dating two weeks when I had to go back to school. It was awful. I think I cried all the way there. I felt like I was leaving part of myself behind. We didn't have cell phones or e-mail back then. We promised each other that we would write every day. We did. I have a shoe box of letters from my wife. She has a much nicer box full of my letters to her. Letter writing is a completely lost form of communication, and it is a shame. I love the fact that I have a written testament to our young love.

I graduated pharmacy school, and Sheryl and I were now a state away. I still lived in Old Bridge and only had a New Jersey pharmacy license. Moving to Pennsylvania was not an option at that time. We had a long-distance relationship, but every weekend I had off, I went up and spent with her. We were so in love that we booked a place for our wedding reception without being officially engaged.

That all changed on August 19, 1995. It was the weekend of our two-year anniversary, and Sheryl had bought tickets for us to see *Phantom of the Opera*. I had another plan. Our movie was *Sleepless in Seattle*. At the end, Tom Hanks and Meg Ryan finally meet at the top of the Empire State Building. I knew immediately after that closing scene that I would ask Sheryl to marry me there.

We left Old Bridge that Saturday morning and took a train to Madison Square Garden in Manhattan. As we were walking toward the theater district, I said to Sheryl,

"It's such a gorgeous day. Let's go up to the top of the Empire State Building."

"I don't want to be late for the show."

It was 11 a.m. The curtain went up at 2 p.m. "We have plenty of time. C'mon, let's go."

It took about an hour but we finally got to the top. We took a lap around and Sheryl was already headed for the elevator.

"C'mon Sheryl, I want to see one more thing." I took her to the east side, facing the harbor. I looked her in the eyes and said, "Sheryl Lynn Harris, when I'm with you I feel like I'm on top of the world."

"That's nice."

"I'm not finished yet." I got down on one knee and presented a ring box. "Will you marry me?"

She welled up with tears and accepted as I put the ring on her finger. As I got up, people were clapping. It was a Hollywood moment, one I will never forget.

On September 21, 1996, (my Mama and Pop's wedding anniversary), Sheryl and I were married. It was right out of a storybook from the perfect weather to the string quartet, French horn, and trumpet playing Handel's "Water Music" throughout the ceremony. Thanks to Mr. Kaschak (my high school band teacher and I'm proud to day my friend) I had the perfect soundtrack picked out.

During the ceremony, we went to give roses to our parents and my Pop, who by the Grace of God, was still going strong at 86 years old. (He would die a year later at 87). He gave us the sagest yet simplest advice. "You be a good husband. You be a good wife."

When my parents were interviewed for the wedding video, the videographer asked them a question: "Do you have any advice for the new couple?"

Dad paused for a moment and thought really hard. "Keep your mouth shut. Walk away once in a while." They were all cracking up. It is the funniest part of the wedding video. By "walk away" Dad meant walk away from a fight. Don't go looking for trouble. Talk about someone who should have taken his own advice.

Fourteen years later, Sheryl and I are still together. Is it all wine and roses? Not even close. We have struggled in various ways as a couple. We have always managed to come out stronger for it. Thank you, My Sweetest Sheryl Lynn, for never giving up on me. I am the luckiest man in the world.

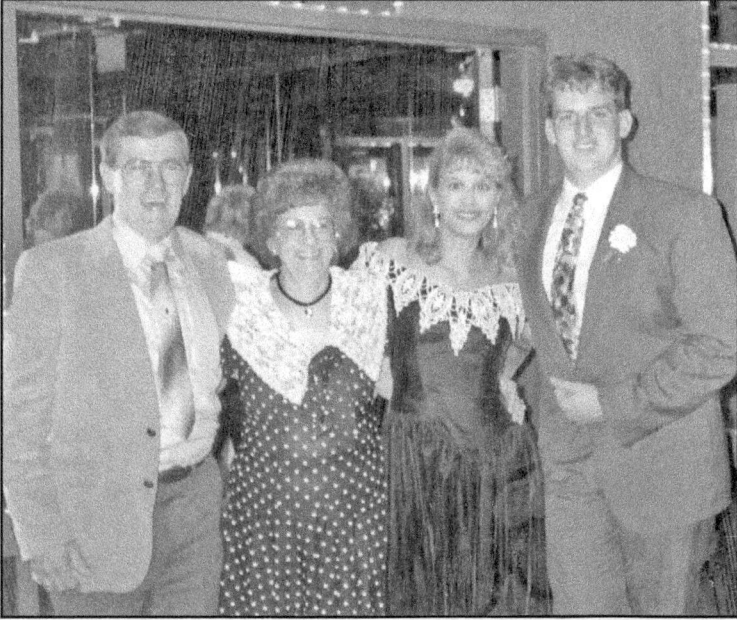

Dave, Frani, Sher and me about two months after we met.

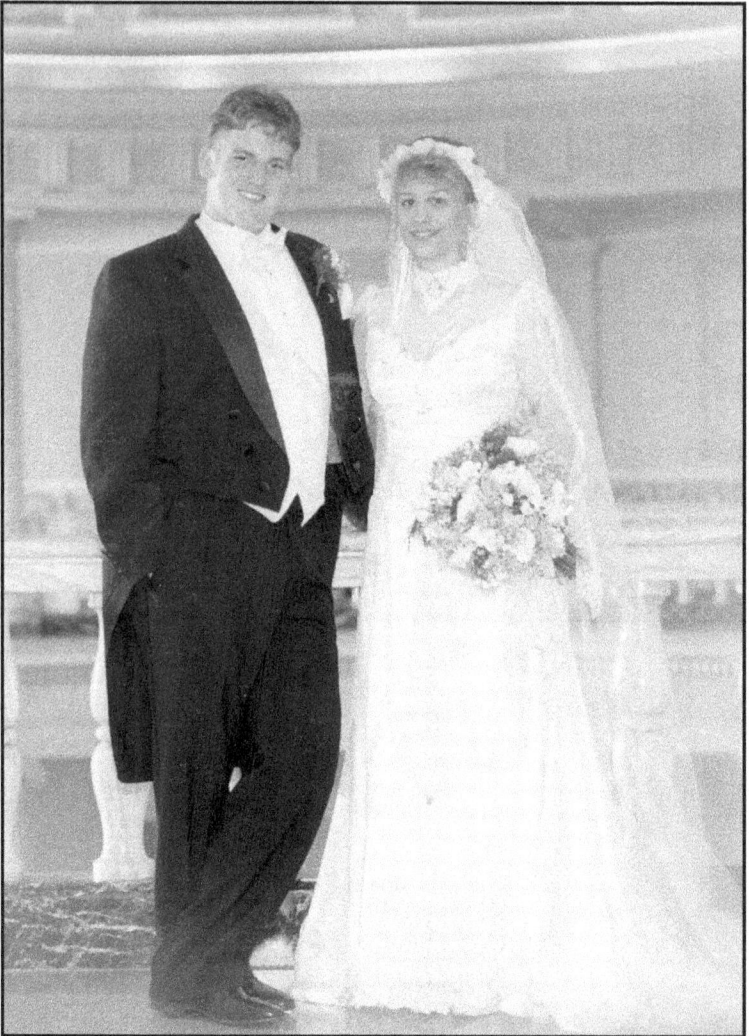

Wedding Day, Marywood Rotunda
"The One"
September 21, 1996

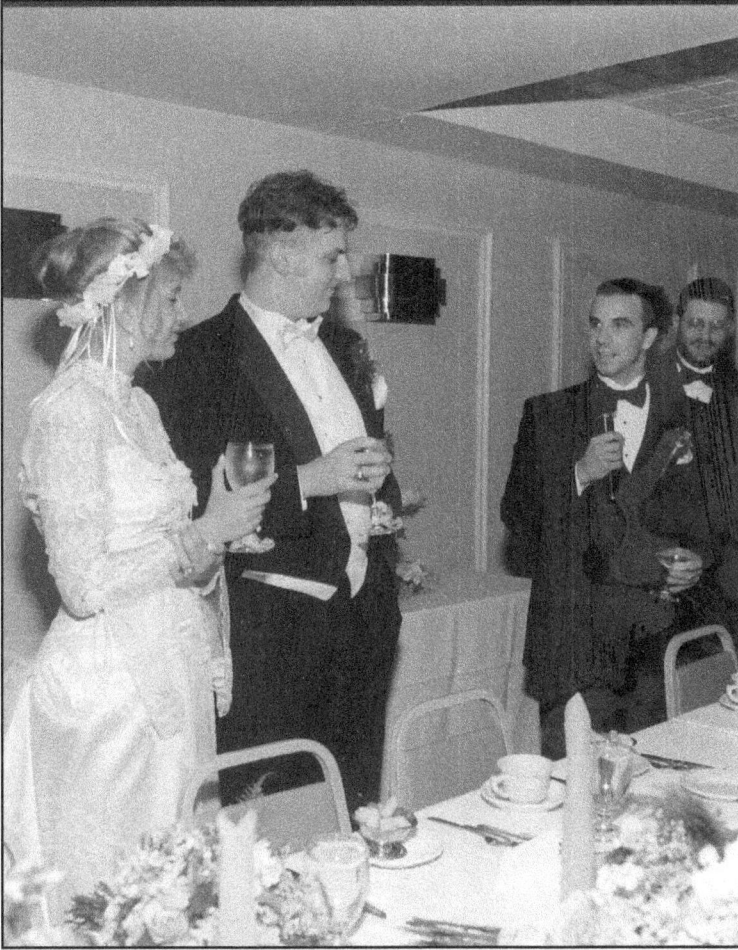

Glenn (holding microphone) giving the Best Man's toast
at our wedding, Sept. 21, 1996

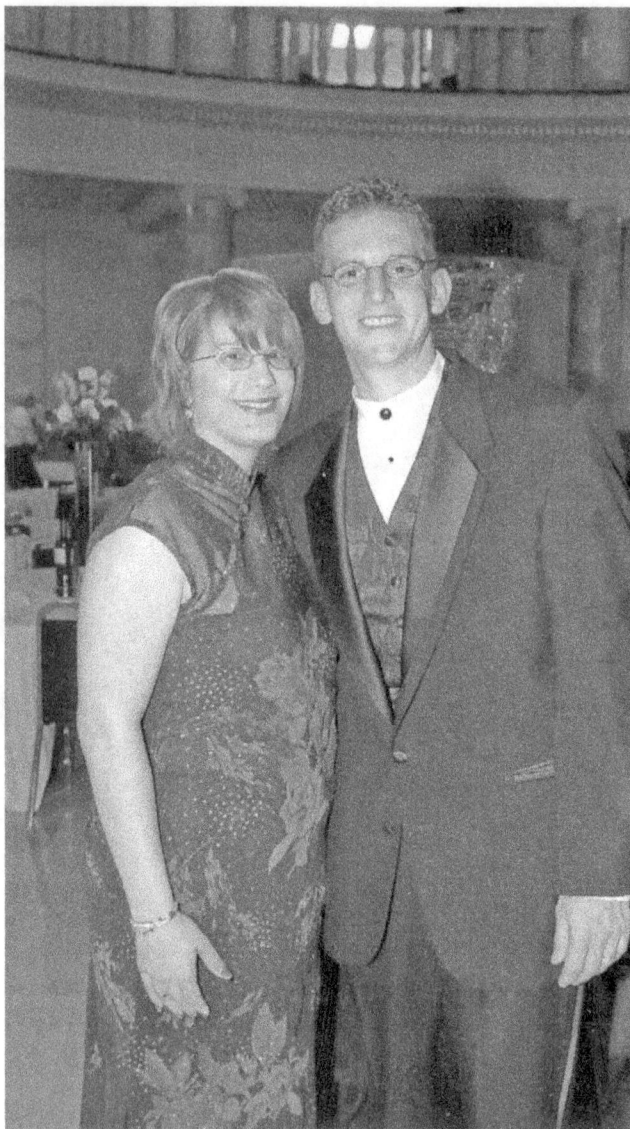

The wife and I
Marywood University
October 2003

8

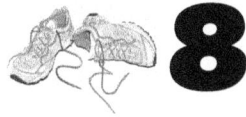

"That's all I can stands and I can't stands no more."

I AM an eater. I love to eat. I eat for pleasure, and I eat for sport. I don't like feeling full. I like feeling gorged. There are three things I know: 1) Foodwise, there is no such thing as too rich. 2) There is no such thing as too sweet. 3) No matter how full you are, there is always room for a piece or two of cheesecake.

Do I eat when I got nervous? Never. I am at my least hungry when I am nervous. It is one of the few times I can say that I am not hungry. I don't eat when I'm depressed, either. I have been known to take comfort in food, though. As a very insecure child, it was nice to take comfort in something.

My wife's family is Italian, and they make the best sauce (not gravy) in the universe. Frani and Sheryl are true masters of tomato sauce. As a friend of mine put it after eating it, "It was Julliard." The Italians and Slovaks have one thing in common. We don't love food, we celebrate it. Seconds? Mere child's play. Try thirds and maybe fourths. When the Olive Garden has the never-ending pasta bowl, they lose money on me.

I once ate two pounds of penne marinara in one sitting. The reward was one free dinner a month for a year. Let's just say that it was a very good year. The scary thing is that I did it in about 20 minutes.

I don't eat one cookie, I eat the bag. I don't eat one scoop of ice cream, I eat the whole half-gallon. I eat really fast, and it takes a lot of food for my body's full buzzer to go off. They say it takes about 20 minutes for that to happen. In 20 minutes, I can eat a whole cheesecake. I never had it officially diagnosed, but there is no doubt in my mind that I have an eating disorder.

With my wife and I sharing the cooking duties, it was detrimental to the waistline. Probably my knees, heart, and back as well. My wife and I both love food. We loved it so much that she had gained some weight, and I was in trouble after four years of marriage.

The title of this book is a bit misleading. I wasn't on the brink of obesity. I was obese. I probably would have been diagnosed "Morbidly Obese" but I was hiding from doctors at the time.

On Christmas Eve 1999, I was playing Santa Claus for the kids at my aunt's house. I grabbed a pillow to stuff in the suit. I could not fit the pillow between my belly and the waistline. I didn't need padding in the suit. I was fat enough. My cousin Michele and I had a laugh about this, but on the inside I was crushed. I thought to myself, "I gotta do something about this."

That night, my wife actually managed to get a picture of me. I was mighty camera-shy back then. I didn't want to know what I looked like. When I saw the photo, I was devastated. I did not even recognize myself. I could not believe how fat I was.

I vowed to do something. It was January 3, 2000, and I got on the scale at my gym. I weighed 306 pounds. I had to lie down on the bed to get my gut to fall in so my pants could zip. I didn't need pliers to pull the zipper up, but I was close. I was trying to fit a 47-inch waist into 42-inch pants.I couldn't believe how much I weighed. I knew I was fat. I figured I went about 275. When I broke "3 Bills" I was heartbroken. I had really let myself go and let myself down. I felt like crying. Somehow, I did not.

"That does it!" I said to myself. "I'm going to do something about this right now!" I had to. I was a disaster waiting to happen. My knees hurt from standing up all day, my back was sore from carrying my belly around, I was a hypertensive heart attack waiting to happen, and more than likely pre-diabetic. I also forgot to mention something. I was also a pack-a-day smoker. Disaster was an understatement. I was more of a catastrophe.

I decided that I would keep going to the gym. I was at the gym often but I did not watch what I was eating. This turned me into a very strong fat guy. Now I was going to watch what I was eating. This time I was going to make my stand. I lost six pounds in my first week, and I was thrilled.

I was so thrilled that, almost immediately, I began slipping up. If there is such a thing as food addiction, and I believe there is, I was relapsing. I stopped watching what I was eating. I would watch and then not watch for months. I managed to not gain weight but I wasn't losing, either.

That April, my family and I took a trip to Disney World. Walking around those parks just about killed me. My wife took a picture of me lying down on a tram station bench. I would see the picture about a week later and it would reinforce the problem that I was fat. I was laying face down in the picture and when I looked at it I thought, "What is that thing under me? OH MY GOD IT'S THE REST OF

ME!" I could no longer hide my fatness by wearing a button down shirt over a t-shirt. I could no longer hide my chins by turning my head a certain way. I was fat, and I felt utterly hopeless to do anything about it.

Then God intervened. He showed me a sign. Not a sign from Heaven but a sign on my gym's billboard. It read, "Weight Watchers, May 19." Weight Watchers? I remembered Weight Watchers. I had been a lifetime member of Weight Watchers since I was 13 years old. Lifetime Membership is when you reach your goal weight and keep it off for 6 weeks. I did this when I was 13 and again when I was about 20. The problem was that as soon as I lost the weight, I stopped following the diet plan. To only my surprise, the weight came back.

There were Weight Watcher meetings in Scranton (I moved to the Moscow Area shortly after I was married), but those 10 miles just seemed too far to drive. The gym was a half-mile from my house. I had no excuse not to go. I walked into the meeting on May 19. It was packed. I was in good company. I got on the scale and weighed 288 pounds. I had managed to somehow lose 18 pounds without really trying too hard over five months. I felt good about that and imagined what I could do if I really tried.

I was introduced to this new Weight Watchers plan with the *POINTS* system. It was this ingenious method of measuring the serving size, calories, fat and fiber of any food and through a nifty slide-rule, assigning a point value to it. The beauty of the plan was that ANY food, in the right serving size, could be eaten. The question was whether the hefty point value of a junk food was worth burning up all of your points on. The *POINTS* system is ingenious and revolutionized the way food is kept track of. That is why they still use it today. The exchange program was good for its day, but it was just too restrictive for me. It did not fit my everyday life. The *POINTS* System fit like a glove.

I had to learn some good habits in a hurry. I had to weigh and measure everything I put in my mouth. I was always heavy-handed when it came to estimating portion sizes. If a serving of meat was the size of a deck of cards, I was using the oversized "Old Maid" cards from when I was four years old. I needed to write down all I was eating in a food journal and subtract the *POINTS* down to zero on a daily basis. If you don't eat the minimum required amount of food, you can actually put yourself into "Starvation Mode" and your body will hold onto the weight. I never had a problem reaching zero. I had to drink a minimum of six eight-ounce glasses of water a day. This does two things. First, you feel fuller, and, second, it helps detoxify your system which, when you are heavy, is very toxic. I also needed to get in 20 minutes of exercise five days a week. I put this off in the beginning. One step at a time. I also shelved the idea of quitting smoking right off the bat. I needed to battle only one demon at a time.

I have to admit that I felt hungry for pretty much the entire first week. I always felt like my stomach did not have enough food in it no matter how much water I drank. I felt like I could have used an extra 10 *POINTS* a day easily. I resisted the temptation to eat more, though. I was also choosing my *POINTS* wisely. I was eating fruit instead of candy. Instead of snacking on junk, I ate the surprisingly low-point sweetened breakfast cereals with 2 percent milk. I could not work my way down to 1 percent or skim milk. I weighed, kept my food diary, and measured to the letter and it paid off. I lost 13 pounds in the first week. I was absolutely thrilled. I got my five-pound ribbon and first five-pound star in the first week. I knew there was a lot of water weight involved, but it still felt good to lose that much weight. For every pound I lost, I imagined what a pound of butter looks like. A pound of butter is pretty much a pound of pure fat. Thirteen pounds of butter could cover a lot of bread.

My success was short-lived. The next week was Memorial Day weekend, and I partied it up for three days. I knew it wasn't going to be a good week on the scale, but I went and took my lumps anyway. I wound up gaining only half a pound. I was pretty happy with that. I may have been knocked down but I got up, dusted off, and continued the fight. I didn't gain an ounce throughout the rest of my journey to goal weight.

Besides your lifestyle modifications, there is a very important part of the plan that needs to be followed. Meetings. Going to meetings puts you in touch with a Weight Watchers leader. The leader is someone who has been in your shoes and crossed the finish line to make Lifetime Membership. They inspire and teach very important lessons to help you stay on track. Michelle DelPrete, I can not thank you enough for all of your help. As a former leader, I never saw a person who just weighed in and skipped the meetings make their goal weight.

What I like about Weight Watchers is that it teaches you how to live. You do not eat three meals and two snacks of flash frozen pre-packaged food. I don't care how fancy their commercials are, they do not teach you how to live. What are you going to do, eat their food for the rest of your life? I doubt it. You are going to go back to doing what you did and put the weight back on. Weight Watchers teaches you self-reliance. You learn how to prepare healthy meals and develop key lifestyle modifications that you can use for the rest of your life. I still keep track of my *POINTS*.

When I added some exercise to my routine, I earned more *POINTS*. The more I worked out, the more I was able to eat. Talk about motivation. I started off easy. My first two exercises were 20-minute brisk walks and playing nine holes of golf while carrying my clubs on my shoulder. The walks got faster and further a little more each week. Over time, I became a power walker. It was summer, and I was spending all of my free time at the lake. I made it a point to get in the water and swim every day I was there. I believe swimming is the best exercise on the planet. It is cardio and full-body resistance training rolled into one.

I was on a weight loss tear. Because of my work schedule, I weighed in every two weeks. I always showed a loss on the scale and wasn't always the model student. On the Fourth of July, I didn't just eat the salad. I enjoyed everything the barbecue buffet had to offer. I ate to the point of supreme fullness. Here is what I did differently. On the fifth of July, I was back on the program. I did not turn the holiday into a holiweek, holimonth, or holiyear. I "got back on the stick" and kept moving forward.

During my voyage, I was blessed with some tremendous news. On September 3, 2000, Sheryl got a great birthday present. We both did. Sheryl was pregnant! I was going to be a DAD! This steeled my resolve to be successful. I did not want to be a couch potato while my child was running all over the place. I wanted to be an active father. I never wanted my kid to see me as fat. I wanted to be in shape for the birth in May. I wanted to be a role model for my child.

Since I wanted to be a role model, I needed to do something else. I had to quit smoking. I could not have my kid see me with a smoke in my hand. Immediately after hearing about the pregnancy, I started a cigarette taper. Over a month I went from a pack a day to nothing. Did I use a patch or pills? No. I substituted something for the oral fixation not replacing one drug for another. I "smoked" some "curiously strong mints." Instead of lighting up, I would pop three Altoids in my lower lip (like a wad of chewing tobacco) and took big diaphoretic drags on them. I would exhale with the pleasure of hitting a butt. It worked. I still do it when I want to have a smoke.

So there I was. Eating under control, no smokes, and now hitting the gym like a fiend. Instead of hating the gym, I was now looking forward to longer and more difficult workouts. I was balancing cardio with strength training. It was shaping me up nicely. In fact when Sher and I went to visit some relatives in California, they didn't recognize me from the last time they saw me. I wasn't at goal weight but I was a good 60 pounds lighter. That's a lot of butter.

While I was good with the weights, I was becoming a cardio machine. I was going for 45 minutes walking at 4 miles an hour with the treadmill jacked up to a 15 degree angle. It was getting to be easy.

Then a voice, which was not mine, said the magic word. "RUN!"

"What?"

"RUN!"

"I don't run."

"Now you do! RUN!"

I dialed up the treadmill to 6 miles per hour. That was a 10-minute mile. I started to run. I also started to feel out of my league. I watched the blips on the treadmill light up one by one to make a complete quarter mile oval. "Just one lap," I said to myself. "Hang in there! You can do it!" The voice was right. I COULD do it! The lights went all the way around the oval. A QUARTER MILE! I DID IT! I was thrilled. I was also panting like an overheated dog so I dialed the treadmill back down to a walk. From then on I would throw occasional ¼ mile laps into the walk. I built up to ¾ of a mile walking to ¼ mile of running. I couldn't believe what I was doing.

It didn't end there. Soon ¼ mile became a ½ mile. Then ¾. I then hit the magic mark. ONE MILE! It took about a month. I hadn't run a mile since being forced to in high school. Somehow I was becoming a runner. I didn't know how this was happening. I gave a lot of credit to being 306 pounds. I was schlepping that weight around for years. That put a lot of stress (not in a good athletic way) on my heart. As the weight came off the heart's ability to move the weight was still there.

Since the weight was gone I could move faster and longer than I could when I was heavy. Due to this, I was able to pile on the mileage.

One mile became two; three and four came and went to my entire five-mile routine being done as a run. I COULD RUN FIVE MILES AT A TIME! I ran so hard that I would trip the breaker on the treadmill! People in the gym were astonished with my progress. "You should run a marathon," someone suggested. I dismissed the idea and stayed happy with my FIVE miles. I would, however, file the idea away and consider it in the future.

December 6, 2000. I crossed the finish line. I got down to my goal weight of 204 pounds. I actually weighed in at 201. I practically back flipped off the scale. That night, I had my wife take a picture of me in the suit I wore on Christmas Eve 1999. I got in the pants, and it looked like a weight loss commercial. I hadn't been at an ideal weight since my third year of college, and that did not last long. I didn't stay on the program back then. This time it would be different. I would stay on program for life. I committed to that statement. That year, I even lost weight throughout Christmas right into 2001. The Santa suit needed a full-size bed pillow in it.

When I got to my goal weight, I treated myself to a new wardrobe. The only new thing I bought myself up to that point was a new belt. I had to buy new everything. Shirts, jeans, underwear—you name it. I went to get my suit taken in, and the tailor said there was no way he could alter the suit to fit me. I had lost too much weight. Talk about coming full circle! I went from being a second grader in the husky section to being turned away from a big and tall shop.

"But I'm tall," I said.

"You're not THAT tall. Go shop at the mall." It was the best money I ever spent.

I was running like a steam locomotive right into February 2001 when a potential disaster occurred. My gym closed down. I was horrified! "Oh NO! NOW WHAT?!" I was still too lazy to drive to Scranton on a daily basis to work out. I had no idea what I was going to do.

"Run outside," the voice said. "You can do it."

I was a bit skeptical. I have heard the ground was unforgiving (it didn't bounce like a treadmill), the terrain was steeper, and, in early February, the weather was most certainly a factor. I live in the North Pocono region. Old Man Winter lives two houses down from me. It was, however, the only shot I had to stay in shape. I marked off a five-mile loop in my truck (the first loop I marked was exactly five miles. There is no such thing as coincidence). I dressed up in two pairs of sweat pants, a hoodie, and a pair of winter gloves.

I went after my first mile, which was uphill and into the wind. It hit me like a freight train. It was COLD! I pressed on. I got over the first hill, and I felt pretty good. Running with a jacked up treadmill perfectly simulated the hill. I was then treated to my first downhill run. It was magical: just that feeling of effortlessly gliding down the hill. It felt so natural. So...right.

I kept moving into miles two and three, then four. One mile from home. I knew I could finish it. Before I knew it I was at my doorstep. I HAD RUN FIVE MILES OUTSIDE! I was astonished but I really shouldn't have been. "Through Him all things are possible." I know who that voice in my head was. It was, indeed, the Lord. I believe that God talks to everybody. It's how you listen that makes the difference.

Along with the running I DID start going to Scranton to hit the gym. I worked out at Marywood University because my wife worked there so I got to work out for cheap. Not only did they have a gym, THEY HAD A POOL! I was able to swim for an entire hour. I was going to reach my goal of really being in shape for when my child would be born.

Through all of this running, I was up to nine miles at a clip in May of 2001. I then made a promise to myself. I dusted off that suggestion and decided to run the 2002 Steamtown Marathon. That story will continue, but now we have to look at something far more life changing. Becoming a Dad.

EVOLUTION FROM

#1
My Pop
and Me
1997

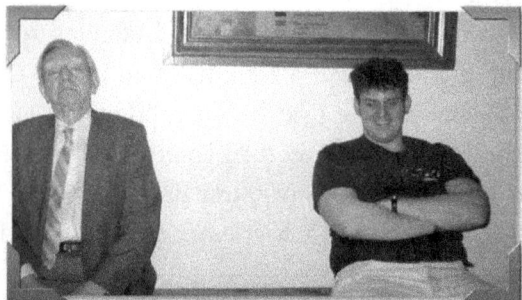

#2

80s Party
L-R Glenn Vignola,
Me, Bob Gilmartin
May 1993

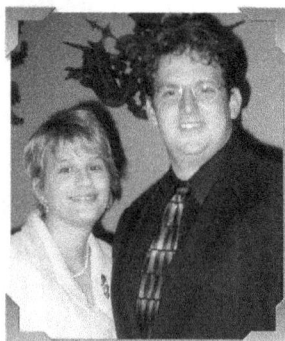

Maximum Density 306 lbs.
Christmas Eve 1999

#4

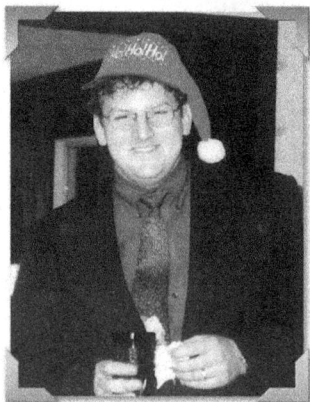

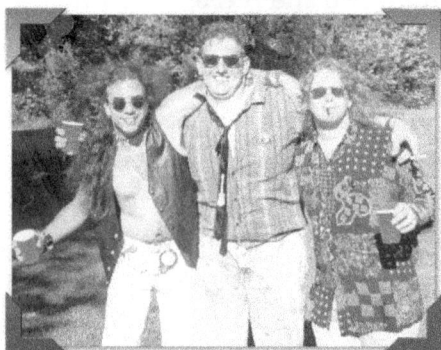

#3   Suit with a
47-inch waist
Aug. 14, 1999

FAT TO FIT

#5 The "Oh my God it's the rest of me" photo April 2000

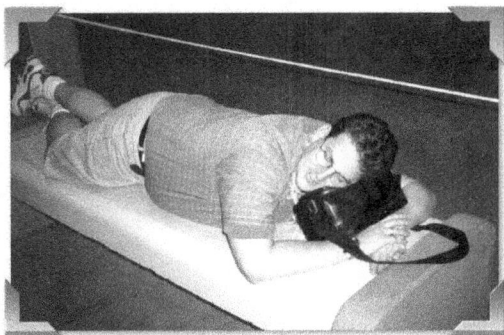

#6 Wife and I at KISS concert Lost about 30 lbs. July 2000

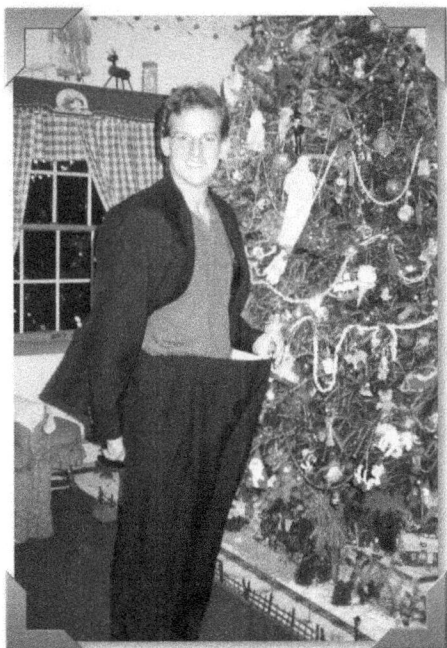

#7 Goal Weight! It's the same suit as the Christmas Eve photo! Dec. 6, 2000

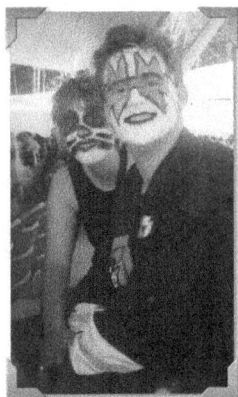

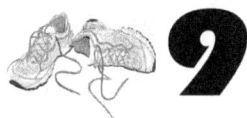

My Child

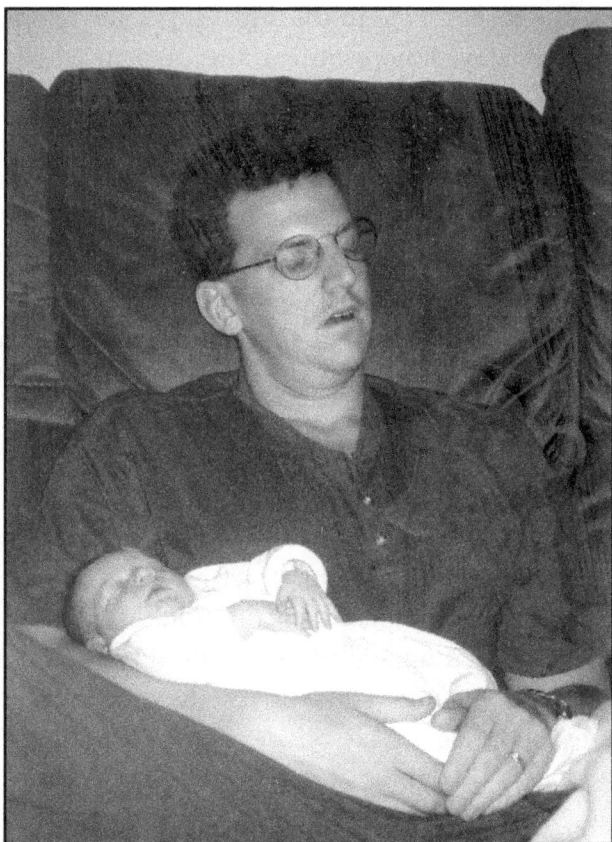

*What do they say about falling asleep
with a baby in your arms?*

Mꜱ AY 13, 2001.

It was Mother's Day. Sheryl and I were kind of bummed that the baby hadn't arrived, but we hosted a dinner for Mom and Frani. We had Chicken Cordon Bleu, and after the company left, I had the mess to contend with. Sheryl was due any day, so the clean-up was all on me.

"I'll do it later," I said to myself. I was tired and needed a nap. The dishes were in the sink and weren't going anywhere. They stayed there until around 10 p.m., when a voice in my head said, "Wash the dishes."

So I did, and was back in bed by 11.

The next voice that woke me was Sheryl's.

"Ohhhhh," she groaned, followed by a sharp, deep breath. I grabbed my watch. The breathing went on for about a minute and stopped. Five minutes later, it came back. Textbook labor. We waited an hour (as instructed), then called the hospital and the OB/GYN on call told us to wait an hour, then come in if it was still happening. It continued. We grabbed the packed bags and headed for Moses Taylor Hospital.

Ask anyone who knows me, and they will tell you I live my life with a continuous soundtrack playing. I basically have a set list for every moment in my life. On the eve of my 30th birthday, I loaded up a jukebox at a local bar. I chose "The End" by The Doors to be the final song. It cued up at three minutes to midnight. The soundtrack for Sheryl's ride to the hospital was NFL Films' "The Power and the Glory," featuring the narration of the late, great John Facenda, who came to be revered by football fans as "The Voice of God." Sheryl was less than pleased with the selection, but we were at the hospital in 15 minutes, so the torture was not drawn out.

I forgot the directions of the birthing class, which were to go to the upper level of the parking deck and get buzzed right in. I parked on the lower level and made Sheryl trudge her way into the ER. She survived, but to this day, she has never let me live it down.

We already had the names picked out: Evelyn Grace (you already know Aunt Evelyn; Aunt Grace is Sheryl's favorite) if it was a girl. Julian Paul was our choice for a boy. I didn't want a Jay Jr., but I wanted to continue the "J name" pattern. From Judy and Joe came Jay. From Jay and Sheryl there could be a Julian. Julian is a derivative of Judy and Paul was my Pop's name.

We had names.

We were at the hospital.

We were all set to go.

Almost.

About a week before the birth, I had a dream that Moses Taylor was booked up and we had to deliver the baby at Community Medical Center in Scranton. The dream turned out to be a vision. When we arrived at the birthing suite, we were told rooms were all full. We didn't have to go to CMC, but we did have to labor in the family waiting room until a post-partum room could be set up for a delivery. I think this freaked out a few of the other family members waiting with us.

In about a half hour, we were moved into a "Mom/Baby" room. The doctor examined Sheryl. "The cervix is ripe," he said. "She's going to deliver."

Soon, we were moved into a birthing suite. It was mid-morning, and Sheryl opted for some pain medication. She put off the epidural and first went with Stadol. This shot sent Sheryl (who never did a drug in her life) right into orbit. The next CD was Pink Floyd's "Dark Side of The Moon." my all-time favorite. Sheryl drifted off to sleep with it playing in the background.

A few hours later, Sheryl's pain increased and she opted for the epidural. When it came time to push, something was clearly wrong. She pushed for three hours, and the baby refused to come. By this time, Frani and Dad were at the hospital.

The baby was stuck. Normally, a baby is born face-down. This one was "sunnyside-up," as one nurse put it. Had the child been face down, Sheryl would have delivered about two hours earlier. Watching the fetal monitor, I could see that the baby was in no distress. Sheryl, however, was exhausted. She said that she could feel her life force draining from her body. Had this been 100 years ago, I probably would have lost them both during the birth. Thank God for modern medicine. It was 6 p.m., and Sheryl opted for a Cesarean Section.

The anesthesiologist came in and prepped Sheryl. She called him "A gift from Jesus." She was then carted off to the OR. I got changed into scrubs, had a quick conversation with the family and went in to see the birth of my child. Sheryl was already cut open when I walked in. They didn't want me to see what was going on until the last moments, so they had me behind a drape talking to the anesthesiologist when he gave me the nod.

"If you look over, you can see the head," he said.

I took a peek and there was a baby's head, red as a tomato, sticking out of my wife. I was about to become a Dad. A moment later, I heard the high pitched whine of a baby crying.

6:48 p.m., May 14, 2001

"This one's male flavored," the doctor said, showing me the baby with face and nether regions facing forward.

"It's a boy?" I asked. "Julian!" I instantly began crying joyful tears. My eyes are welling up as I write. Julian Paul Sochoka had finally arrived. I had a son, which I expected all along. Here's why:

It was August of 1997, and Pop was on what would become his death bed at Mercy Hospital (the third hospital in Scranton). He was talking with Sheryl. He was really out of it for most of the time, but had occasional moments of clarity.

"Are you knitting something?" he asked Sheryl.

"Why would I be knitting?"

"For the baby," Pop replied matter-of-factly.

"There's no baby, Pop."

"There will be."

Sheryl indulged him.

"Will it be a girl or a boy?"

He looked upward, deep in thought. The answer came. "A boy."

Back in the OR I said, "Pop was right, Sheryl! Pop was right!"

Julian was weighed, measured, and fitted with an ID bracelet. Then the nurse asked, "Do you want to hold him?" He was minutes old and so fragile, but I was not afraid to pick him up. My arms knew exactly what to do.

I brought him over to Sheryl, who was too out of it to really appreciate the moment.

"Can I take him to the family?" I asked.

"He's yours. As long as you stay on the floor you can do whatever you want," the nurse said.

I left the OR and walked right across the hall in to the room. With Julian and a video camera in my arms, I entered the room singing, "Hey Jude."

"It's a boy, Dad," I said. He really wanted a grandson.

His arms shot up into "the touchdown sign."

"Woo Hoo Hoooo!" he cheered.

We were in the hospital from Sunday to Friday while Sheryl healed up. In that time, I gave Julian his first baths, changed his first diapers and held and walked him around the floor for hours on end. I would sing to him two things—a lullaby I wrote for him and "When I'm 64" by The Beatles. It had a nice tempo to walk to and gently bounce him with as I roamed the hallways in the early morning hours. It knocked him right out. I was referred to as "Daddy Ether Arms."

It's nine years later, and I am still in awe of the whole thing—the learning to crawl, walk, and talk; his ridiculous intelligence; the things he comes up with that make me laugh to the point of tears. There is nothing he could do to make me love him less and nothing else he could do to make me love him more. He's everything to me. I would give my life to save his and, as I tell him all the time, it is very cool to be his Dad.

Thank you, God, for bringing Julian Paul into my life. Thank you, Julian Paul, for completing it.

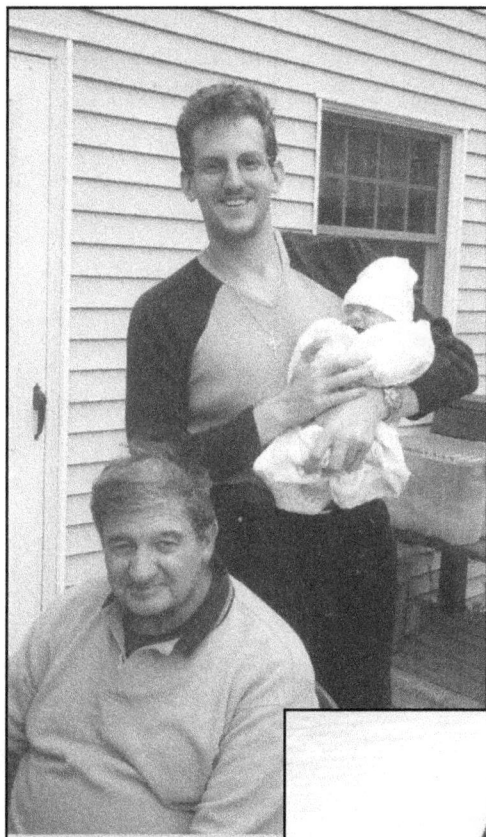

*Three generations of
Sochokas on my first
Father's Day, 2001*

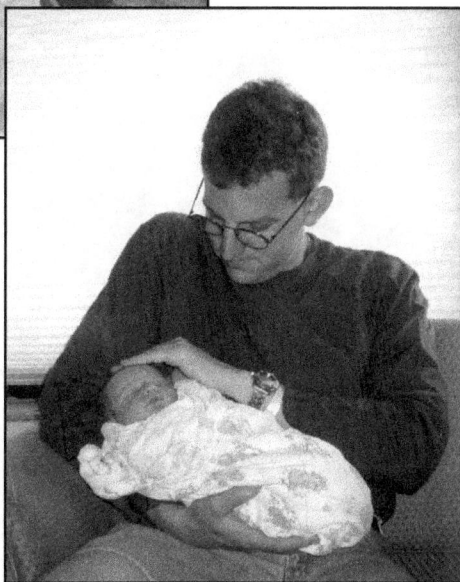

*Julian and Daddy in
the hospital. Julian
was two days old.
May 16, 2001*

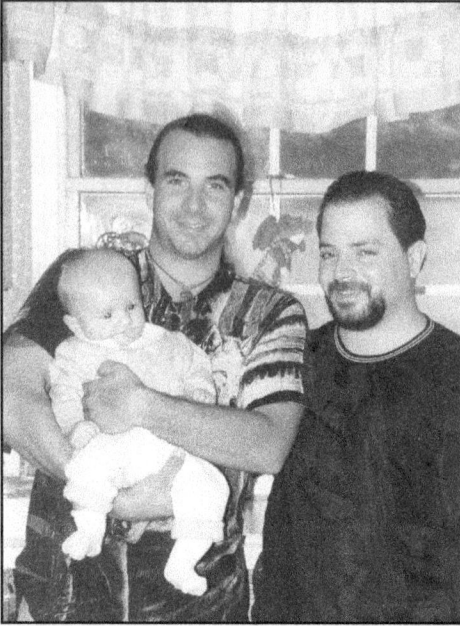

Julian, Uncle Glenn and Uncle Joey

My family, Newton Lake and my boat. What more could a man want? July 3, 2007

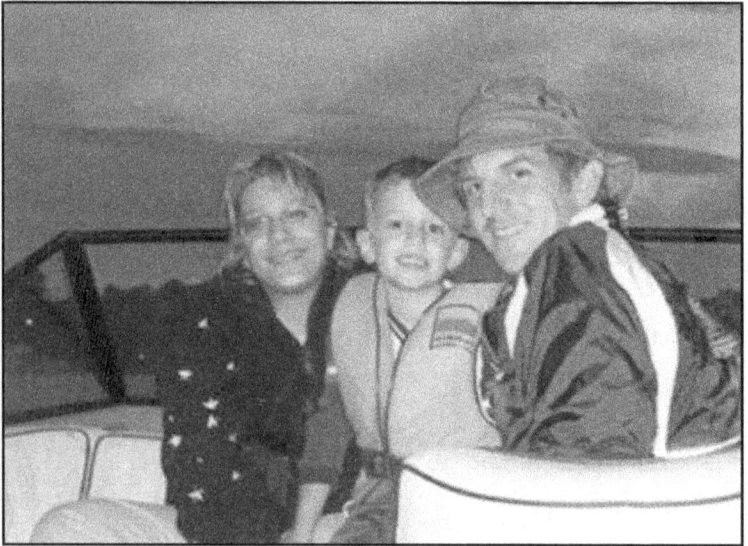

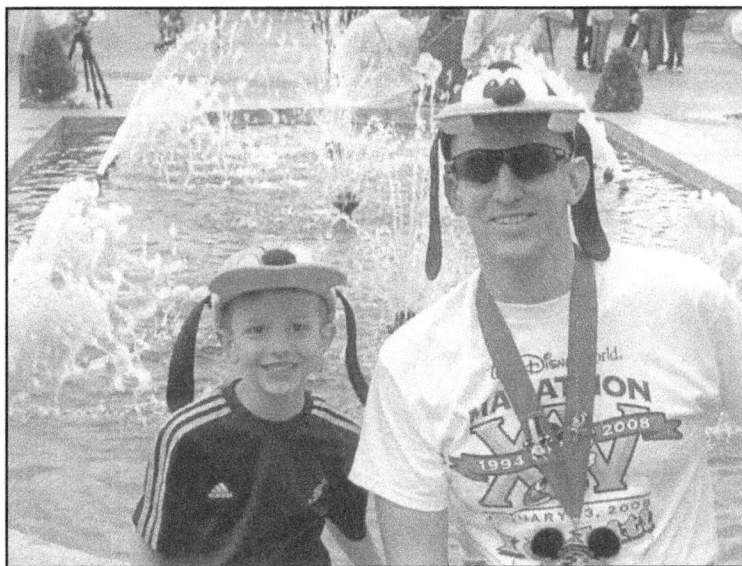

It can be said that I'm Goofy for my son

We're all a bunch of kids at Christmastime

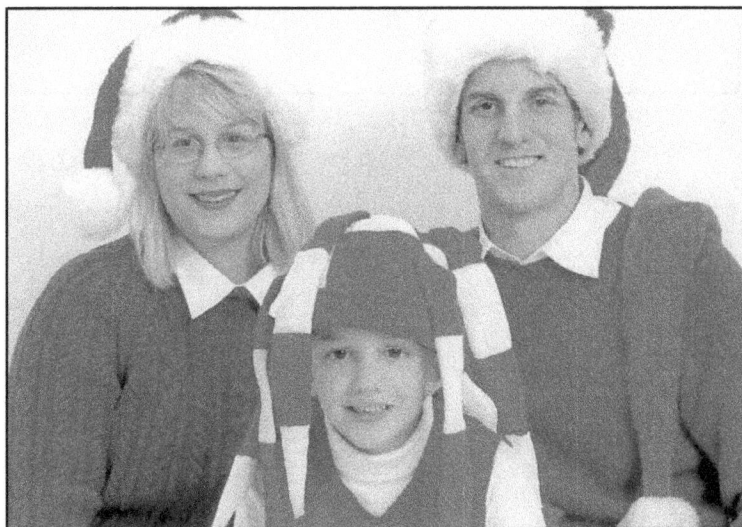

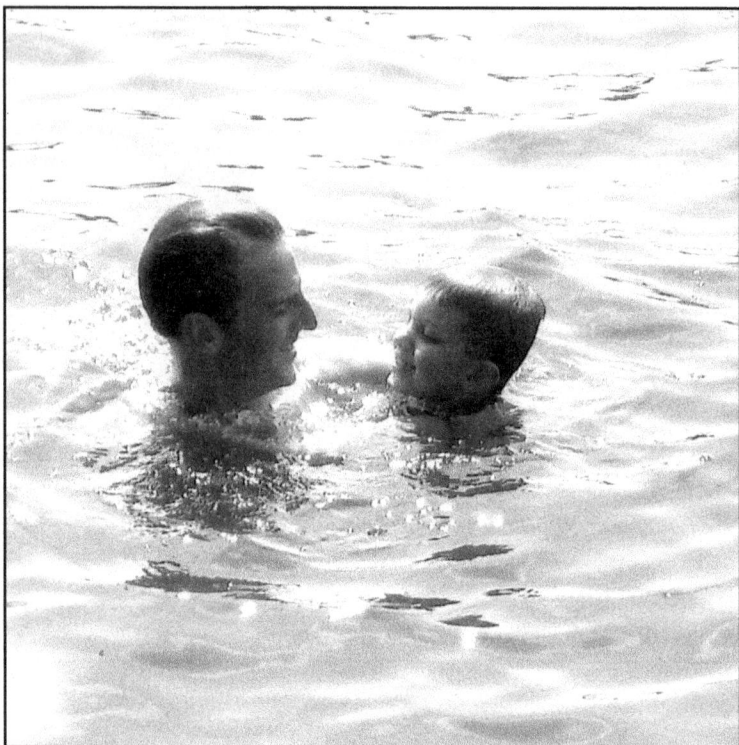

"It gets no better"

10

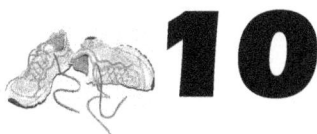

My First Steamtown and What I Learned From It

MY running had really progressed through May, June, and July. I was able to do a long run of 16 miles. I had a resting pulse of 38 beats per minute. I knew this, because I had to undergo some medical testing; I would pass out and hit the floor when I urinated.

They were able to rule out epilepsy, which was originally suspected. It turns out I had what was called micturition syncope. When I woke up in the middle of the night to pee, my heart rate was around 30 beats per minute. That led to a really low blood pressure. When I relieved myself of some liquid volume, my blood pressure would bottom out, causing me to faint. At least we got to the bottom of the problem, and it was not epilepsy. The treatment was to sit on the bowl if I had to do number one. I was relieved. Pun intended.

I was talking to a friend of mine who had run the Steamtown Marathon. Her name is Michelle Lacoe, and she was one of those "crazy marathoners" I used to shake my head at as I drove by. I told her I was planning to run the 2002 Steamtown Marathon.

"What's your long run up to?" she asked.

"Sixteen," I replied.

"You can run Steamtown this year," she said. "Just get up to 20 miles and you are all set."

I trusted her and registered to run the 2001 Steamtown. I could not believe that I was 306 pounds in 2000 and was going to run 26.2 miles in 2001. It was incomprehensible to me.

It was July, and I decided that I should do a race before running the marathon. Forest City, PA, hosts "The Coal Cracker 5-Miler." I had watched this race from the sidelines for years as I kid. I never in my mind thought I'd be a participant. I registered, warmed up, and got on the line.

BANG!

The pistol didn't scare me this time. The pack took off. I made the near fatal mistake of chasing it. I came across the one-mile split in 5 minutes and 48 seconds. While it was the fastest mile I had run to date, I was way out of my league. When you race, remember this lesson: Go out comfortably, get into a groove, and then pick off people throughout the race. It is a much smarter way to run. It is also more satisfying to reel people in than get passed by everyone. The latter happened to me for the next four miles.

I had to slow down. There was no way I could keep going at that pace. I survived the race and managed to run it in 36:14. I ran so hard then when I stopped, I almost blew chow. I was fighting for my life, but I had done it!

I wasn't alone when I ran it, either. Mom Dad, Sheryl, and Julian went with me. The first three cheered for me as I came in. Julian slept through it. It felt good to have a few fans come out and cheer.

This brings me to August tenth. My 30th birthday. I had achieved a milestone. It was my goal to get in shape before I turned 30. I was in the shape of my life. It was a runner's birthday party. I was given running clothes, a gift certificate for high-end sneakers, and the coveted runner's watch. I was now able to time how long I would be out running. I used to look at a clock when I started and when I finished and estimate my time. I was really just building up my running base. I had never even heard of speedwork.

Soon after my birthday, I ran 20 miles one week and 23 miles the next. I was told not to exceed 23 miles and to leave the last three for the race, making your first marathon the longest run of your life. It would make it just that much more meaningful. Since I reached my limit, it was time to start tapering back down. This gives you time to rebuild your legs so you are fresh for the race.

Before I knew it, it was Columbus Day Weekend. The 2001 Steamtown Marathon was here. It was 5 a.m. the morning of the race, and I was up like a shot. Excited was an understatement. Nothing gets me out of bed at 5 a.m. I didn't even know that 5 a.m. existed. I had breakfast, and my wife drove me the five miles from my parents' house to Forest City High School.

Fifteen minutes before the start time, I took a position in the middle of the pack. It is good race etiquette not to get in anyone's way. Bishop Timlin blessed the field. I was grateful. I needed all the help I could get.

Then the national anthem was sung. September 11, 2001, was a month earlier. The attacks were very fresh in our heads. We were asked to wear patriotic colors. I actually made a uniform that had blue shorts with white stars and a vertical red and white striped top. There were American flag shorts and red, white, and blue ribbons all over the place. I never heard "The Star Spangled Banner" sung with more emotion. I don't think there was an American runner in the field who wasn't singing.

It was time to get going. The race was started by a Civil War Reenactment Brigade that brought a cannon. The race director got on the microphone. "Runners ready. Runners set."

BLAM!

The cannon went off and so did we.

Running through Forest City is an awesome experience. It was 8 a.m., and the people were out in force cheering for us. They rang the church bells as we ran by. At the one-mile mark, the high school band played us out of town. One down, 25.2 to go. I felt great, and hoped it would hold up.

Mile 2 starts a very generous downhill portion of the race. The running feels effortless, and it's easy to get ahead of yourself. Somewhere around Mile 3 a voice rang out.

"Is this your first marathon?"

"Yes."

"Get behind me," the voice said. "You are running seven-minute miles." His name was Marty, and I could not thank him enough for his advice. I couldn't believe that I was running so fast. It was just too easy. How did he know I was running seven-minute miles anyway?

As we crossed another mile marker, I saw many a runner press a button on their watches. "What are they doing?" I asked.

Marty answered, "They are pushing the split button; it breaks up your miles into individual parts."

Five miles into the race, and I learned something new. My watch had a split button. From then on I "split" my miles. Before I knew it, I was at the halfway point: 13.1 miles at around 1:38. I had set three goals for this race:

Finish it. To finish is to win.

Run it in under four hours.

Run it in under 3:30.

If I could hold on, I could break 3:30. My legs were starting to get sore. At Mile 14, I met up with Sheryl to grab a water bottle and a gel, which is like cake icing filled with sugar, electrolytes, caffeine, and amino acids. It gives the system a nice jolt when it kicks in. She gave me a thumbs-up as I went by. As I passed her I saw a runner who was not as fortunate.

A female runner was on the curb standing next to an EMT and was crying. Her race was over. My heart broke for her. I wanted to stop and cry with her. I felt awful. It could be me there. There but for the grace of God go I. I pressed on, set my eyes forward and kept going. I still had a job to do. I rounded a corner and the terrain changed.

We were now on the Rails To Trails part of the course. This is absolutely beautiful to see, but it is torture to run. With the Lackawanna River on one side and peak foliage on the other, it is easy to get lost in the moment. The terrain is tough, because you don't bounce like you do on the road. You sink into the trail. While it is a nice rest for the legs, you have to run harder to keep up your pace. I was spending all the energy I had and getting slower every mile. I wasn't worried about finishing under 3:30. I was worried about finishing.

At the 20-mile mark there is a naval war memorial with an anchor from an actual ship sitting there. In a marathon they call Mile 20 "Hitting the Wall." I call 20 in Steamtown "Carrying the Anchor." I felt like I was dragging that anchor all the way to Scranton, a good 3.5 miles away. This is the part of the course where it starts to go uphill. The toughest part of the race has the toughest terrain.

I crossed Mile 21 and observed the casualties piling up around me. Runners were walking. Runners were limping, Runners were holding their butts or stopped and massaging their own legs. We were also entering the no-man's-land part of the course. No bands, no cheerleaders, no crowd; just a landfill at the 22-mile mark to see. I knew that Sheryl was a mile away for the last handoff. I needed her bad. I was hurting.

I trudged to Mile 23 and saw her. "Almost there, honey! Keep going!" I was 3.2 miles away from finishing my first marathon and facing the dreaded "Electric Street Hill."

At the bottom of the hill, a huge sign says "Welcome to Scranton." It is there that the race's most rabid fans gather. They absolutely roar for you. It makes the tough climb a lot more bearable. In the middle of the hill, you cross Mile 24. 2.2. At the top is a school called St. Joseph's Center. It is for the severely physically and mentally handicapped. The race benefits the center, and students line up to show their appreciation of the runners. The sight moved me to tears.

And then it hit me: I was about to finish my first marathon. "You got this," an inner voice said. "You are going to finish."

He was with me. God wasn't my co-pilot, he was my running buddy. He was with me and he was going to carry me home. I knew without a shadow of doubt that I would finish the race. I looked at my watch, and I also saw that I was going to break 3:30. I was elated.

I ran down Capouse Avenue and made the left toward Washington Avenue, where the finish line was, and crossed mile 25. *One-point-two and home,* I thought. I rounded the corner and saw a mountain in front of me. I had forgotten that Washington Avenue had a hill twice the size of Electric Street in the middle of it. The only consolation was that I knew the finish line was on the other side. I climbed the hill and got to the Masonic Temple. The mountain turned from sheer cliff to gentle grade. Before I knew it, I was over the top and could see the finish line.

Just past mile 26, in front of City Hall, something else caught my eye. It was Mom, Dad, and my cousin Michele. Michele took my picture as I flashed the "V" for victory sign. Mom gave me the V sign back. Dad. Dad was clapping and cheering his head off. The look on his face said it all.

"There goes my son. The natural-born athlete." I never saw him so proud of me.

Final time: 3 hours 24 minutes 32 seconds. I had finished. The fat kid who finished dead last every time he ran a lap at soccer practice had finished his first marathon. To finish was to win, and at that moment nothing felt impossible.

Here is what I learned from running my first marathon.

Nothing is impossible. If you put your mind to it and work really hard, you can (within reason) do anything you put your mind to. When it comes to an idea, If you conceive it and you believe it, then you can achieve it.

Run your first marathon without a watch. Enjoy it, don't time it. You have the rest of your life to worry about how fast you can run a marathon and set personal records.

It is easier to walk stairs backwards than forwards after a marathon. In fact everything from my neck down hurt. When my shoe untied, I could not bend down to tie it. I had to ask someone at work to do it for me.

Take the day after off from work. I realized this after it took me half an hour to put my pants on. Like I said, everything hurt.

Three things: Believe in yourself, believe in yourself, and believe in yourself.

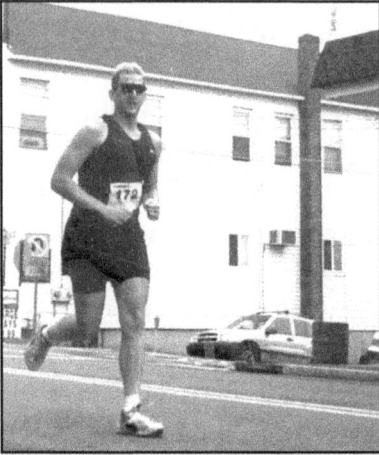

Warming up for my first race as an adult
Coal Cracker 5-Miler
Forest City, PA
Aug. 2001

Home Stretch
Finishing chute
of my first
marathon

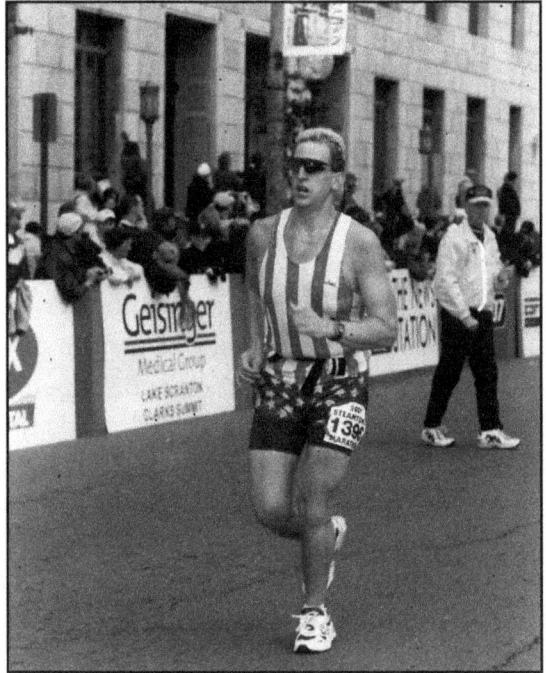

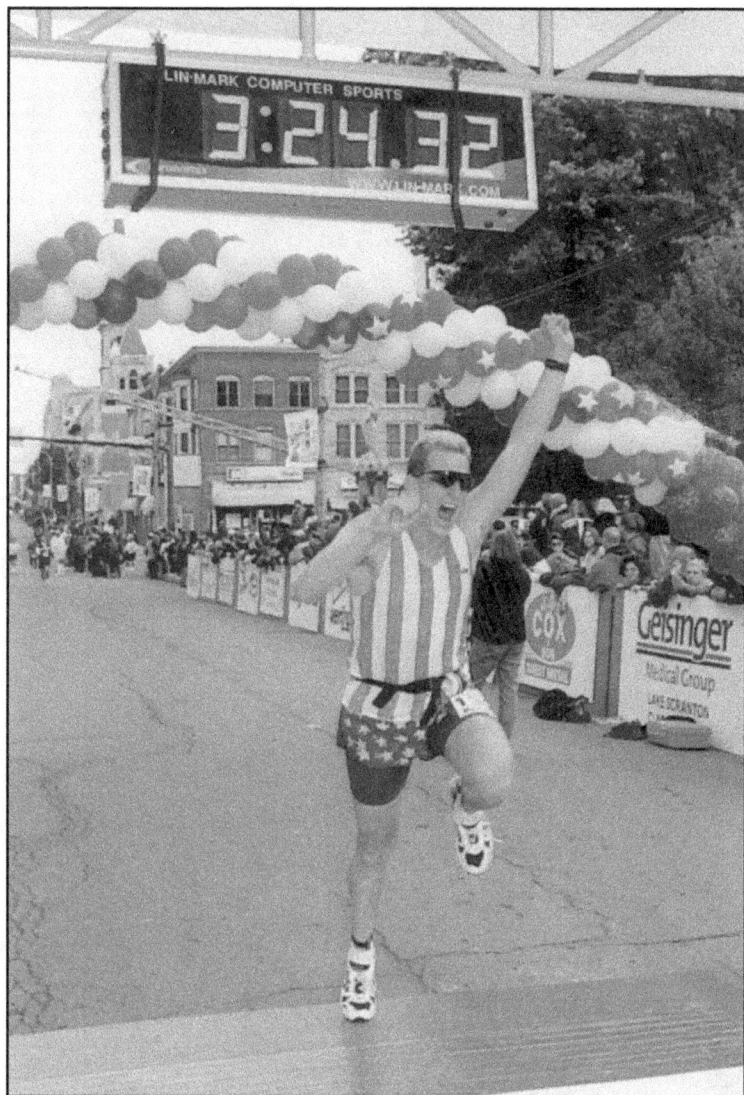

Steamtown Marathon
Scranton, PA
2001

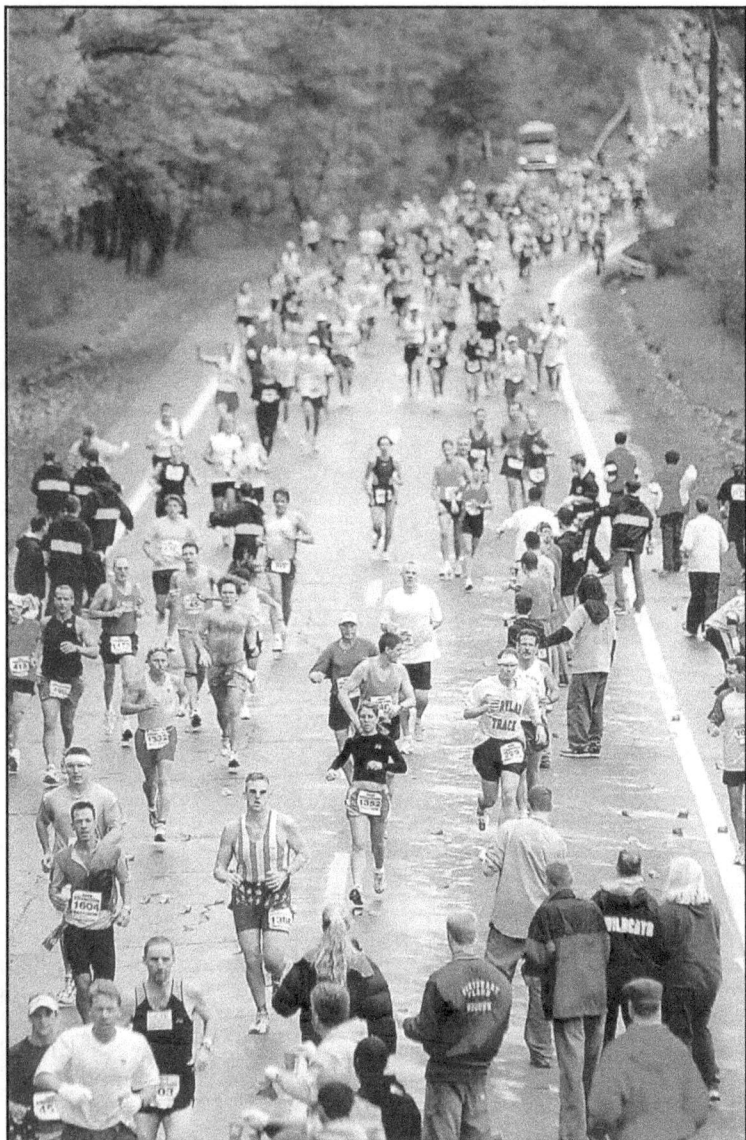

Can you find me?
An awesome photo taken by Butch Comegys
of the Scranton Times-Tribune
Steamtown Marathon, Oct. 8, 2002

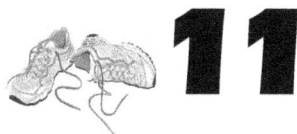

11

Dad Gets Sick

I N July of 2000, Dad had given us quite a scare. He was complaining of chest pains and was rushed to the hospital. He had a mild heart attack. We thought he had dodged a bullet and was given a second chance. It turned out to be the beginning of the end.

At the 2001 Steamtown Marathon, Dad stood and cheered for me. When I ran it in 2002, he was sitting in a chair and stood up to take my picture. In 2003, Dad watched me finish Steamtown Marathon from a wheelchair.

Dad had a hand tremor since 1995, when he was put back on lithium for his bipolar disorder. The neurologist chalked up the tremor to the drug. As a pharmacist, I knew this was a side effect so I didn't think twice about it. It was harder to ignore the fact that Dad was getting noticeably weaker.

"I'M GOING TO THE GYM, AND I CAN'T LIFT WHAT I LIFTED LAST WEEK!" he screamed at Mom during a fight. I wondered why he was getting so mad over the natural aging process. It turns out his decline was more rapid than simple aging, and it was scaring him. When you get that scared, you get angry. He was afraid and taking it out on those closest to him. It's a trait I know all too well.

Mom took Dad to his physician, and he was diagnosed with Parkinson's disease. Mom wasn't happy with the answers she was getting in Northeastern Pennsylvania so she went down to Philadelphia to the Hospital of The University of Pennsylvania. She figured Philadelphia doctors might have a better idea of what was going on. They didn't. While they were sure Dad did not have Parkinson's, they could not nail down what it was. "Unspecified Neuropathy" was what they called it. Mom had to have a better answer, so she kept looking.

It was at the University of Medicine and Dentistry in New Jersey (UMDNJ) that the verdict was handed down. It was a death sentence. Multiple System Atrophy. I had never heard of the disease before. I soon found out why.

In pharmacy school, they only teach you about diseases that can be treated pharmaceutically. Why didn't I hear about this disease? It's simple. There was no drug treatment for it. The doctor suggested trying one of a handful of anti-Parkinson's drugs available called amantadine. It actually made his tremors worse.

At the time, I was becoming a very strong runner. I was able to run over 30 miles at a time on a whim and Dad was losing his ability to walk. As I grew stronger, he was fading away. And there was nothing I could do to help him.

Here I stand with no less than a million dollars worth of pharmaceuticals at my disposal and not one could help Dad. Not one! I could give an 80-year-old man the thrill of his golden years by giving him a blue, diamond-shaped pill at $15 a "pop," but all the money in the world could not buy Dad an extra second on this Earth.

MSA has been described as getting Parkinson's disease, Multiple Sclerosis, and Lou Gehrig's disease all at the same time. Having witnessed what happened to my Dad, I'd say it's too kind a description. He was given 4-6 years from the onset of symptoms, and after some research on MSA, I knew much of that time would be spent in pain and fear.

MSA starts its work in the central nervous system, then branches out to the eyes. It affects the nerves of the bladder and intestines, causing incontinence. Eventually, it paralyzes the muscles of the throat so swallowing is impossible. Finally, MSA attacks the respiratory system and paralyzes the diaphragm. Dad would die of respiratory failure, and I would have a front row seat.

I wish I could say that caring for Dad came naturally and was the easiest thing I ever did. That would be a lie. It was didn't feel natural at all, it was the hardest thing I ever did.

It was hard for two reasons: First, it killed me to see Dad decline so rapidly. I would go to the lake to let Mom go out on Fridays and just get away from it all for half a day or so. At least it gave her a little break. For purely selfish reasons, I hated going.

Every week I went there, something was worse with Dad. I gave him a ton of credit, though. He didn't ask for my help unless he absolutely needed it. I was watching TV in the living room as Dad was getting dressed in the adjoining bathroom. I could hear him cursing under his breath. I knew what was coming next. "Jay, could you help me get dressed?" Without saying a word I went in there and put clothes on my Dad. Julian was a toddler then, so I was pretty good at dressing him, and I just tried to look at it that way. It didn't help any. When I finished dressing him, Dad said, "I'm sorry."

"Don't be," I replied. "You did this for me when I needed help. Now I'm helping you." I hoped putting it that way would cushion the blow and it seemed to help.

The second reason it was hard to take care of Dad was the bad blood that lingered between us. Did I love him? Absolutely. But the fact of the matter is that in my lifetime he said and did things to Mom and me that were absolutely despicable. There were times when I felt that he was an evil monster. There were times I wished him dead. Be careful what you wish for huh?

So when it came time for me to take care of all of my Dad's bathroom needs, I was resentful. I felt like Dad was now paying the price for his past. He had it all coming to him. Sure, Dad was going to get to Heaven, but he was going to have to go through Hell on Earth first.

It turned out that he felt the same way. He told Mom that God was punishing him. I felt awful when I heard this. I know that this is not how God operates. It is, however, exactly how The Enemy gets you to think. When he gets a hold of your thoughts, bad things can happen. My thoughts were pure poison. I needed help. My wife saw this need and called a counselor for me.

John Lemoncelli, Ed.D. was a psychology professor at Marywood University with a private practice. His reputation for dealing with children of abuse was, and still is, stellar. When I called for an appointment, the secretary told me that his book was quite full for the foreseeable future. When Sheryl made the call and used the Marywood card, I got in the next week. Thank God.

John is a man of deep faith. He uses his faith and a belief in a higher power to heal his patients. In his book, *A Mind of Its Own: Healing the Mind and Heart of the Parasite of Childhood Abuse* (Avventura, 2008), John likens the results of childhood abuse to a parasite forming in the psyche. The parasite latches onto your thoughts and contaminates a great deal of them. Like all parasites left untreated, this one will consume and destroy the host. The treatment is simple: No parasite can survive in a host that is anchored firmly to his or her God. It took me years to learn that, and I wish I had known it as I watched Dad drift away.

In times of crisis, people often demonstrate obsessive behavior with alcohol, drugs and the like. I was no different. My drug of choice was running. I would beat myself up for miles on end. I would play the past and future in my head while flying down the road with reckless abandon. I would argue with God while holding down a 7:30 pace. Ten miles would disappear in the blink of an eye. Mom would get home from her day out and I would practically bowl her over getting out the door to score more miles. Qualifying for Boston was all I cared about. I would do whatever it took to get there at all costs. It was all that mattered to me.

That, and what was happening to Dad. I have to give him a lot of credit. He could have been a real bitter bastard up until the very end and no one would have blamed him. He didn't. He reached the acceptance stage with grace and made his peace with God. He lived his life as well as his body would let him. He collected all the memories he could. He might not be able to play catch with Julian, but he could sit him on his lap.

It was Father's Day 2004, and I was chasing Julian around the yard. I looked over and Dad was watching us with a kind of sad look on his face. "How I wish I could chase him," he told Mom. Hearing that broke my heart.

Before I knew it, Columbus Day Weekend had arrived and, with it, Steamtown and my chance to qualify for Boston. I didn't know if I would ever get another chance, so I dedicated this race to Dad.

I needed a 3:10.59 to go to Boston. I ran a PR 3:11.38 and missed going to Boston because of a one-minute stop in the woods. The fact is I didn't care. I ran the race of my life and Dad, who was tough to get around, came out to see me. Crossing the line that day felt as good as the first time did. Pure victory is still there.

The phone rang that night. It was Dad. He never called me. Something was up. "I have to tell you something," he said. "I want you to know how proud I am of you with your running. I'm proud of you, son."

"Thanks Dad," I said. "I know how hard it is for you to get around and I want to thank you for coming out. It meant so much to me."

Silence. Then a sniffle. Oh my God he's crying.

"You take care of yourself," he said. "I love you."

My eyes welling up, I said, "I love you too."

I knew right then that Dad would never see me race again. I'm glad he got to see me at my best. It meant a lot to me.

We enrolled Dad in Hospice when he was first diagnosed. People often wait until the last minute to get hospice involved, and that is a mistake. Hospice is for the terminally ill not just for the obviously dying. They help the patient and the family. They bathed Dad, so I wouldn't have to. They had people minister to him spiritually. They ministered to us. They took a lot off of our minds. They would be there in the end to administer any comfort meds in Dad's final hours so no one in the family would have to get their hands dirty.

As morbid as it is, a funny story arises every time the subject of comfort meds is broached even to this day. Mom was talking to Sheryl, and said, "Hospice came today and dropped off a comfort pack."

Sheryl had misinterpreted the fact that the pack was for the patient and not for the family. "What's in it? soaps? Lotion? Candy?" she asked.

"Uh, no," Mom replied. "Ativan, compazine and morphine. It's for his comfort, not ours."

If you don't laugh in moments like this, all you are going to do is cry.

After New Year's 2005, Mom was exhausted. She was doubting her ability to care for Dad and was debating putting him in a nursing home. Before we took that giant step, we checked him into the hospice unit for a three-day respite. That would give us time to think about what we were going to do next. Hopefully. it would give Mom the strength to keep taking care of him.

I went to visit Dad in the unit one day and noticed that his roommate was dying. His eyes were closed and his breathing was shallow and heavily labored. He was also alone. There was no one with him. Not a family member; not even a nurse. I vowed that this would not happen to my Dad in some nursing home. If I had to, I would move in to help Mom.

The next day, Mom, Sher, Julian, and I all went to visit Dad. To no surprise, his roommate wasn't there. I wonder to this day if Dad knew what was going on. I'm sure he did, but he didn't say anything about it.

We were all talking for a while when all of a sudden Dad looked around the room. "I love you, Jude," he said.

"I love you, Joe."

"I love you, Jay."

"I love you, Dad."

"I love you, Sheryl."

"I love you, Joe."

"I love you, Julian"

"I love you, Pop-Pop"

There was no doubt in my mind that Dad was ready to die. He was saying goodbye. It was only a matter of time.

It was Sunday January 16th 2005 at 9:30 a.m. I just got back from a run, sat down to check some e-mail, and the phone rang. The caller ID came up as Mom's number.

Oh no.

12

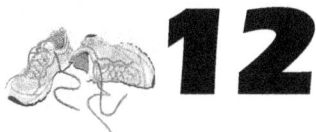

This is the end...

"HELLO?"

The five-second pause before Mom started talking said it all.

"Jay...you better come up here. He's not dead, but I can't wake him up."

"I'm on my way."

Still sweaty from a run, I got out of my chair and got ready to leave. *I need to pack a bag. Wait. No time.* "Sher? It's Dad. He's not gone, but I have to go. Pack me a bag and I'll see you there."

I don't remember much about getting there. I was probably flying. I just prayed to God to keep him until I got there. I needed to talk to him. Something was on my chest that I needed to get off before he died. I needed to make amends.

I pulled into the driveway and sprinted through the door. Mom was downstairs by Dad's hospital bed. We converted the living room to the bedroom. The house was planned that way in case, when my parents got older, they could not make it up the stairs. I never thought we'd have to employ it so early in their golden years. Golden years. That's a laugh. For Dad, it was more like the lead years. Anyway, like Mom said, Dad was unresponsive. I also noticed that his breathing was labored. This was the beginning of the end. He could die today all without my chance to talk to him.

About an hour after I got there, Dad came to. *Oh, thank God. Now is your chance. Do it now.* You might not get another one. With tears streaming down my face I started. "Dad? I need to tell you something. There were times when you were sick that I treated you pretty shitty. I just want you to know I'm sorry."

He was unable to speak, but his eyes answered. He reached up, hands fiercely trembling, and grabbed my hand. With all the strength he had, he moved his lips. I read it as clear as day. "It's OK."

I was forgiven. Right then and there he forgave me. It may have been selfish to focus on that for the time being, but I needed it. I was so grateful to not have to carry that burden for the rest of my life. If you need to make amends with somebody, do it now. You might not get another chance.

Speaking of amends, there was another conflict that needed resolution. My Aunt Maryann (Dad's sister) and Mom had a falling out when I was 13. Imagine the look on my face when she showed up at the doorstep about six months before Dad died. Even with the falling out, it was good to see her. I was always so fond of her. Not to mention that she was a nursing home R.N., so she would be able to tell us what was going on. Mom called her, told her what was going on, and she was on her way.

We also called hospice and they showed up before I knew it. The basic lowdown was that he didn't have "a lot of time." They couldn't tell us exactly how long he had, but they told us he was dying. "Give him his food," the nurse said. "Just make him comfortable."

Sheryl, Julian, and Ralph (our dog) showed up within a few hours. Dad was a bit more with it now. He tried to talk, but his speech was horribly garbled. I was watching a football game. The Giants were playing. "What's the score?" he mumbled. That was the best thing I heard all day. At least he had the wherewithal to know that there was a football game going on.

"21-3 Giants," I said. We watched the rest of the game together. It would be the last time we would ever do that.

It was getting late. I had to work the next day, so I needed to get to bed. I said good night and wondered if it would be the last time.

I woke up Monday and checked on Dad. His breathing seemed a bit more labored than the day before. He was getting worse. I said goodbye and headed off to work. I was in another world. I got to an intersection and almost ran a stop sign in front of a cop. He gave me a stern look and waved me through. Thanks.

I was heading down Route 247 when Chief Fortuner came up behind me. I looked down and saw that I was going 70 mph in a 45 zone. The cherries and blueberries flipped on and I pulled over. It was cold, so he didn't get out of the car. He just pulled up alongside me.

"First you run a stop sign and I let you go," he said. "Now you're going 70 miles an hour on a road with snow drifts. WHAT ARE YOU DOING?!"

"I'm sorry, Chief," I said. "My Dad is dying. I'm staying there and am on my way to work. My mind has been wandering. I'm sorry."

Without getting out of the car he motioned me forward. "Go on, get out of here," he said. "Be careful." I pulled away and somehow got to work without causing a pile-up.

God was good to me that day. As a pharmacist, I need focus in my job. I managed to get through the day without killing somebody. It was nothing short of a miracle, because my head was not in the game.

It was Tuesday, and the rounds of goodbyes had begun. Cousin Paul showed up. He is not the type who wears emotion on his sleeve. He usually hides behind humor in a tough situation. Paul and Dad were close.

"I don't know why I even came up here. You don't look so bad to me!" Paul said. This made Dad smile.

"I'll see you in a few days," Paul said as he left. He was right. He would see Dad at the funeral.

I was off work on Wednesday, so I got to stay with Dad at the lake. I can't remember it being a good day or a bad day. I just remember not going for a run on my day off, which was odd at the time. I always ran on a day off. Rain, snow, ice it didn't matter, I would run anyway. Not that day. If Dad was going to die, I wanted to be there. I can't explain why. I guess I wanted to make sure that he wasn't alone when he passed.

Dad's breathing grew increasingly labored the next day. I noticed. So did Sheryl. Mom didn't want to. There were some very unpleasant moments in their marriage, but he was still the love of her life. She was not ready to let him go.

"Mom, if you want people to come over now would be the time to call them," I said.

"Do you really think so?"

"Yes, Mom. He doesn't have a lot of time left."

Mom called Aunt Maryann, Aunt Evelyn and Uncle

Mike. They must have had their bags packed, because they were there before I knew it. We stayed up and kept an eye on Dad. He was breathing hard, and his eyes were closed. He looked just like his roommate in the hospice unit. It was late, so I went up to bed. We had a baby monitor running from the downstairs to upstairs bedroom. If something changed, I would hear it. I fell asleep to the sound of Dad's breathing. He sounded like Darth Vader running a marathon.

Friday morning came. His breathing was shorter and harder. We thought he would die that morning. I was called down many times to say goodbye. Aunt Maryann was keeping a close eye on the situation. She had a lot of experience with death. We trusted her judgment. When she called me down, I came running. We were encouraging him to go, but he just wasn't ready.

"Jay," Mom said. "Call the priest."

This made it very real. It was time for The Last Rites. I called Father Sitko and got his answering machine. I told him the situation and asked for a prompt call back. It came. "Father," I began, "Joe Sochoka is dying and we would like you to come and give him the Last Rites."

"I'm on my way."

Father Sitko came, absolved Dad of all of his sins, and we began the "Our Father." The first prayer I learned as a child would be one of the last Dad would hear. I'm sure you know the prayer but I'll share with you the unique way it was done at my Dad's bedside. "Our Father (scratch scratch scratch; Ralph was still outside and wanted to come back inside. He was letting us know his business was done and it was cold out) who art in Heaven. Hallowed be thy name. (scratch scratch scratch) They kingdom come (scratch) they will be done (scratch) on Earth as it is in Heaven. Give us this day our

99

daily bread (scratch) and forgive us our trespasses. (scratch scratch) as we forgive those who trespass against us (scratch scratch) and lead us not into temptation (Ding Dong! Yes the dog rang the doorbell to come inside and it took everything in my power to not crack up laughing in such a somber moment) but deliver us from evil. Amen."

Even Father Sitko was stifling a smile. Like I said, if you don't laugh in moments like this, all you will do is cry.

Father finished the Last Rites and we were at ease. Dad was as ready to go home as he was going to get. Father left and we settled in for the end to come.

Dad wasn't done on this planet yet. He still had something he needed to do. He wasn't going anywhere until it was done. We did everything we could to make him comfortable. He was running a ridiculously high fever. We put ice packs on his neck to keep it at bay. We told him it was OK to go, but he wasn't ready.

On Friday night, Dad's eyes opened. He looked around the room and locked his eyes on Mom. He could not talk, but he didn't need to. "The Platters Greatest Hits" was right next to the CD player. My parents danced to the Platters countless times. They would have one more dance; not with their bodies but with their eyes.

When "The Great Pretender" came on, one of the most beautiful things I ever saw happened. Dad locked his eyes on Mom and with all the strength he had left he picked his head up off the pillow and puckered his lips. He wanted to kiss her goodbye.

In that moment, I could see how much my parents loved each other. I had trouble seeing this during their fights. I saw that I was created out of their love. Their love was true. Pure. Undying.

We wanted to give Mom and Dad one last night together, so we put a recliner next to his hospital bed and set them next to each other. They kissed each other goodnight and Dad's eyes closed. Mom was the last thing he would ever see. Dad's eyes never opened again.

I noticed that Dad's finger and toe nails were a mess. I took clippers and trimmed them. I was preparing him for his trip. I wanted him to be presentable when he met The Lord. I know it sounds funny, but it was how I felt at the time. I didn't want him to meet Jesus with dirty fingernails. Neither would Dad. He was obsessive about keeping his nails groomed.

Mom woke up, and Sheryl and Julian came into the room. We dug in for what would be Dad's last stand. His breathing was beyond erratic now. It was a sound I was all too familiar with. It sounded exactly the way I sound when I run up a hard hill. When I run a hill now, I always think of Dad's final hours. There is no way around it.

With the exception of Julian, we were all gathered around the bed. I was on Dad's right and Mom was at the head on Dad's left. We sang Dad's favorite hymn, "Holy God We Praise Thy Name." He wouldn't leave. Aunt Maryann prayed for favor, and we begged God to take him. No go. I leaned in close, put my mouth to his ear and said, "Why are you staying? There is nothing here for you anymore. You have somewhere more beautiful to go. We'll be OK. Go home."

This was going on for hours. It was now 6 p.m. and it seemed like this could go on all night. I gave my Aunt Evelyn a look. It said, "Help me."

She knew what I meant. "I don't think there is anything more we can do for him now," she said. "Why don't we help him?" No sooner had she finished the sentence and I produced the Ativan and morphine that I had grabbed from the comfort pack earlier in the day.

Dad's life had come to the point where these two drugs could help him. Finally, the pharmacist had a job to do.

"I can do it if you want me to, Jay," Mom said.

"No, Mom, this is my job."

Some of you at this point may question my view on the sanctity of life. Let me assure you that I view life as the most precious of God's gifts. From the "glint in the eye" to the final breath, I view life as sacred. Dad was dead except for a small part of the brain called the medulla oblongata. This controls involuntary functions such as heartbeat and breathing. Dad was dead, but that part of his brain forgot to shut off. His quality of life was nil.

I placed two Ativan in his mouth and used about three milliliters of morphine solution 20mg/ml to dissolve it. I'm not an idiot. Morphine in high enough doses will depress the respiratory system. I knew that this was going to stop his breathing. This would, without a doubt in my mind, end my father's life. I gave him another milliliter or two every couple of minutes. I put my ear to his chest.

"If you want to say goodbye," I said, "now is the time."

"Julian, "Mom said, "come and say goodbye to Pop-Pop."

Julian, who was only three years old, walked over and said "Goodbye, Pop- Pop." He then walked back to the television to watch cartoons.

"Goodbye, Joe," said Sheryl, Uncle Mike and my aunts.

"Joe, Baby," Mom said, "I love you, but it's time to go home."

I gave him another milliliter of morphine as we started to sing, "Holy God, We Praise Thy Name." The room was filled with our singing and the sound of Dad's labored breathing. *Don't fight it. Let the drugs do their job.*

Heaving breath...Heaving breath...Heaving breath... Silence. Dead silence.

I looked down at my watch. It was 6:30 p.m. on January 22, 2005.

"That's it. He's gone."

Looking back, his death was beautiful. He was lifted up in prayer, and he was not alone. In fact, he was surrounded by those closest to him. He did not die alone. When it is my time, I hope I am that blessed.

Did I cry when my Dad died? Not a tear. I was too relieved. I truly believed that he was in a better place. I knew his suffering was over. I knew that he was truly home.

On Christmas Eve, we observe the Slovak tradition of taking an apple and cutting a slice for every person at the table. From that slice, we cut a piece for everyone at the table. They do the same. Everyone gets a piece of everybody else's apple. The message is this: If you are ever lost or ever in trouble you think of who you shared the apple with and go to them for help.

We could have let Dad be and let the funeral home take care of him, but it just didn't feel right. Mom got a basin of warm, soapy water and three washcloths. Mom, Aunt Evelyn, and I gave Dad his last bath. It was now time to get him dressed. I vowed that Dad would not wear a diaper when he left the house that night. I looked around and found a pair of briefs. I slipped them over his legs and got them around his waist. We then put a sweatsuit on him. He looked comfortable.

After we got Dad presentable, everyone else came downstairs. Dad's dog, Jesse, lay beside his body and would not leave it. When it came time to take Dad's body away, she began howling and would not stop. Her heart was broken. We said our goodbyes to Dad and left the room. Before I knew it he was gone. I missed him.

The next few days were a blur. Friends and family poured in and out of the house. We had more food than we could possibly eat. I did my fair share of grief eating. There was definite comfort in it.

On the morning of the funeral, we were up around six. I let the dog out. It was the coldest day I had ever felt. The sun was up, but the moon was still in the sky. It was then that God sent us a sign. Mom saw it first. The moon was high in the sky and there was a halo around it in the shape of a cross. It looked like the Host (Communion wafer) in front of the crucifix. The image is prevalent in many Catholic churches. We tried to take a picture of it, but it would not come out. It was meant for us to see and us alone. It told us exactly where Dad was and who would be with us that day. It gave us indescribable comfort.

It was time to say goodbye. I bid farewell to Dad's body at the funeral home. Now, through my eulogy of him, it was time to say goodbye to his spirit. My cousin Michele had a copy of it in her coat in case I was overcome with emotion and could not finish.

Be with me Lord. Here we go.

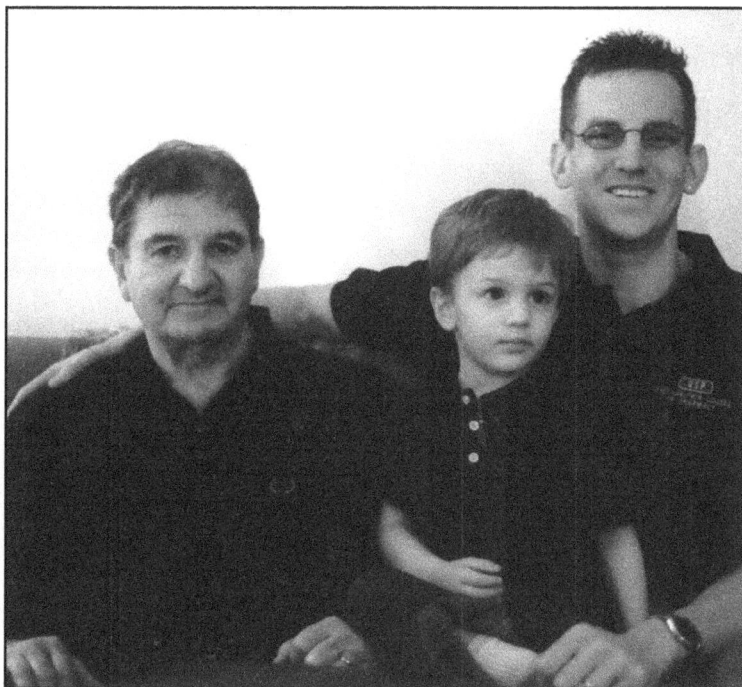

Dad, Julian, Me.
Spring, 2004

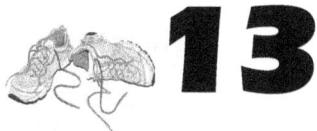

13

Dad's Eulogy

HERE it is, word for word. The parentheses are there to describe a person you haven't met yet in this story.

The Champ: A Tribute to My Dad Joe

My Dad loved sports.

I can't tell you a favorite professional team of his, because I don't think he had one. High school sports were more his cup of tea. He had his finger on the pulse of the Riverside Girls Basketball and Softball teams. Marissa (Riverside High School athletic standout, and our cousin, Marissa Chisdock) , he was your number-one fan.

To be a Sochoka, in this area, meant baseball, football, and basketball were in your blood. It was your birthright to have talent in one or all of those sports. In my life, I played one season of baseball, never put on a football helmet, and to this day can't do a lay-up without hearing someone chuckle.

That never mattered to Dad. After school, we would practice in the field by Schirra School. He would pitch, I would hit. He'd hit pop-ups and I'd catch them...on the forehead sometimes which explained why I wore a batting helmet during fielding practice. We'd play catch and we'd have fun. That is what it was about. Just having some fun with Dad.

I picked hockey to be my sport. Although he was not a true fan of the sport, he came to see every game he could and was there when I scored my one career goal against Beacon Hill. He beamed with pride and I received $5 for my effort. I think he had a feeling my NCAA eligibility would never be in jeopardy. I was having fun and that was all that mattered.

The one sport we enjoyed together was boxing.

Like my one career goal, Dad had one career fight, and if you have ever seen the film of it, you might mistake it for a Three Stooges episode. Paul Yarros was his corner man then, as he was through life. My Dad did not have a lot of friends. To become my Dad's friend, you needed patience to get to know the man under all the barriers. Once you did that, you realized what a terrific person he was.

Back to the boxing. Even though my Dad went 0-1 in his career, he still enjoyed the sport. He thought Rocky Marciano was the best ever, Ali was a bum, and always sighed with relief when a boxer closing in on Rock's 49-0 record would suffer a defeat. Dad taught me to box. In an open space in the house, we would go a few rounds.

When I was younger, he'd fight from his knees and always throw the fight. As I got older, he'd stand up and I had to defend myself. Our last fight ended with an uppercut to his ribs, which knocked the wind out of him. He did not beam with pride at that moment, but he realized he had taught me well. "Use this only to defend yourself," he told me. I listened. In my life I never started a fight. I did, however, finish a few.

The other sports we enjoyed together were at Newton Lake.

The hot days of summer were our favorite. How we loved to eat breakfast by the water, go for a swim, go waterskiing (I skied, he drove, Alice [Newton Lake neighbor and friend Alice Russell] would spot), swim again, spend time by the water, have lunch and dinner by the lake, take a bath in the lake, and, when the nights were warm enough, go swimming again. The big splash heard all the way in the kitchen meant Dad took a dive off the dock. His legacy is our lake house. It was his idea to buy it, and the greatest idea ever had on earth, as far as I'm concerned.

It's no coincidence that Dad died when he did. This is the time when he would head to the warmth of Florida.

He would never leave Newton Lake in the summer.

How I loved to take boat rides with him. As a kid who pulled away from the dock and go full throttle, he showed me the joy and beauty of the slow lap. The quiet time of fishing at sunset, I believe was his favorite time. He caught a few lunkers in his time but he was there just to enjoy the moment. Once again, the end result was inconsequential.

When he retired to the lake, I was so happy for him. Finally, he would be at his favorite place on Earth. Finally, he was back where he wanted to be. After 30 years of living in New Jersey, he was home. We loved Pennsylvania so much growing up, we would lean forward to be the first one in the state. When the toll went one way, he observed, "You can go to Jersey for free, you have to pay to get into Pennsylvania."

Dad led an active life when he moved up here.

Five days a week he was in the gym. He was taking care of himself for when a grandchild came around. "Make sure you have a boy," he told me. I don't think he was kidding.

When I brought Julian from the delivery room and said, "It's a boy," his arms made the touchdown sign, and he cheered. Julian became the apple of his eye and his chance at redemption.

We were not the Bradys. In fact we were more like The Simpsons. Like all families, we said the wrong thing, or got upset, and even had the occasional argument here and there. It took me a long time to realize the demons that were chasing my father. Some all the way from birth. However he would not just say, "That's the way it is, it was handed to me." He fought them tooth and nail.

He'd get knocked down here and there, but he would always get back up. He won many rounds over the years, and although he might have been against the ropes, he never got knocked out or threw in the towel. He fought valiantly and showed me how far he came from where he started.

"I love you," were three words in his vocabulary that he used often. I never felt that it was wrong to kiss my father hello or goodbye, anywhere on this planet. I could never shake my father's hand goodbye; it just would not feel right to me. He showed me how selfless he could be when we bought our new boat. I wanted to go halves on it, but he said, "No, I can swing this, I want you to have it." We enjoyed many rides together in it before he got sick.

My Dad getting sick was the hardest thing to see in my life.

For someone to get sober, quit smoking, watch what he eats, and hit the gym—to have that happen seemed very wrong to me at the time. He got angry, at first. We all did. Then something wonderful happened. Once the anger left, the demons went with it. He made peace with his fate. If you read The Passion, you will remember that Jesus had a fight with the Father before saying, "Your will be done." My father was no different, and his cross was no less a burden.

In his last fight, he fought with courage honor and dignity. He did everything his failing body would allow him to do. He saw all of the Steamtown Marathons I have run. Finally I got to see the "That's my son" look on his face.

I think about it almost every time I run. I will run every race from now on in his honor.

He saw countless high school athletic events, most of which were Riverside softball and Girls basketball. He became the greatest Pop-Pop the world has ever seen. Without a doubt, his mark is left on my son. His love for Julian showed me how much I was loved when I was a boy.

In his last week he fought his final rounds. He was absolutely valiant. He was more concerned for us than he was himself. "I love you," he said to Mom, Julian, and I in the hospice unit. "Are you ok?" he asked my mom in his last days. He embraced visits and calls from everyone in the family, and I want to thank you all for everything kind you have ever done for my father.

On Friday, we knew the end was soon, and we called Father Sitko. As you all know, my father loved to crack jokes and break up a quiet room with a gag or two. Therefore, I find it no coincidence that while Father Sitko was giving last rites, my dog Ralph rang the doorbell because he was cold. It was a joke that was right up his alley.

On his last night, I realized why my parents were married. They loved each other like no two people I have ever seen. I put the Platters on the stereo and watched my Mom and Dad dance the night away. My Dad said his last words with his eyes, and they were, "Judy, you are the love of my life." It was one of the most beautiful things I have ever seen. I will cherish it forever.

I will also cherish the way my father left this earth.

I'd be up here for another hour if I tried to explain it to you. For those of us who were there, it was a life-altering experience. Ask me about it and I will tell you sometime.

I want to thank my Mom for taking such terrific care of Dad. Like I said that night, you are extraordinary. You are the reason that Dad was in such good shape for as long as he was. The level of care you gave him was like nothing I have ever seen. God gave you all the strength and peace you needed to handle such a burden.

To everyone at Hospice, especially Michelle, Dawn, Joe, and Iris. (Michelle and Dawn were nurses. Joe gave pastoral care. Iris was his aide): One million thanks. You started out as our caregivers. You became our friends.

To everyone in our family: Thank you once again for all you have done.

Today, we say farewell to a father, a husband, a brother, an uncle, a cousin, and a friend.

I, for one, will miss him but I am so happy for him. He can walk, his hands don't shake, and he is at peace. I will miss him, but I take great comfort in the fact that he is having such a great reunion in Heaven right now.

The 15th round is over. The final bell has rung. It's time to hang up the gloves, Champ. God Bless you.

Jay J. Sochoka, R.Ph.
January 25, 2005, 8:41 p.m.

When it was over, St. Pius X church came alive with applause.

"I have been doing this for 20 years, and I never heard a eulogy that beautiful," one of the funeral directors said.

That felt really good to hear.

Dad was to be cremated, so there was no trip to the cemetery. Good thing. The weather was still brutally cold. Instead, as the crowd left the church everyone grabbed a rose and laid it on his casket as "Holy God, We Praise Thy Name" was played for him one last time.

Now the tears came. The outpouring of love shown for my Dad overwhelmed me. I was finally able to feel something. I was sad because I missed him, yet so glad that he was in a better place. I know I will see him again. In the big picture of eternity, it won't be that long a wait.

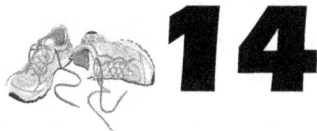

14

A.D.
After Dad

MY Aunt Maryann hit the nail on the head. It was about three months after her father died when it hit her. Her Dad was gone. He wasn't coming back. She was driving her car and had to pull over. She was inconsolable. The same thing happened to me, only it took me two months.

It was the Sunday after the St. Pat's Parade in Scranton. I had spent the day before getting pretty torn up with Bob Gilmartin and a bunch of my running buddies. We had a really good time. Probably too good. Definitely too good. I was up way too late and when Sunday came around I had gotten about two hours sleep. I felt plenty rested though. We'll get to why I felt that way later. Since I felt so good, I went for a run then went to church.

I was sitting in a pew at St. Eulaila's (my home parish) when during the offering the organist started playing "Hosea" which is probably my favorite hymn. The organ part is full of beautiful arpeggios and the words are equally such. The line came. "Long have I waited for your coming home to me and living deeply our new life." It hit me like a cinder block. I started crying and had to do everything in my power not to all-out sob. The Mass ended, and I high tailed it out of there. I cried all the way home.

Bob and I then picked up where we left off on Saturday. Dumb idea. I did not need to throw booze on top of how I felt. It just added fuel to the fire. I was laughing one moment and crying the next. Then it hit me.

"I killed him, Bob."

"Who?"

"Dad. I killed my father."

"No, you didn't. You helped send him home."

"NO, BOB! I KILLED HIM!"

Bob did his best to try and talk me down. It didn't matter. I cried the whole afternoon. Bob had to go back to N.J., so I kept it going with Sheryl. She assured me that I helped Dad. It sunk in that she was right, but I still missed him. It all of a sudden hit me that I would never see him again. Because of this, I could not stop crying.

Eventually, I did, and I managed to sleep that night. I woke up the next day, and it was like it never happened. I guess I had gotten it out of my system. While I still miss my Dad terribly, that never happened again.

Meanwhile, I had taken my training to a new level; 26.2 miles didn't feel like a challenge anymore. I had decided to go Ultra. Not only was I going to run further that I could ever have imagined, I was going to do it for charity. I had decided to do two runs to raise money for children's Miracle Network. CMN raises money for children's hospitals all over the country so that no child is ever denied the life saving treatment they require. They pick up where insurance leaves off. If the family doesn't have insurance, they pick up the tab. If you are ever feeling philanthropic, send them a check. It is a wonderful organization.

While I had committed to the runs before my Dad died, there was a reason on the day my Dad died that sealed the deal. My friend Chris DiMattio and his wife, Ann, had a son Louis Carlo, in mid-January. There was a problem; his aorta was malformed and he needed life saving surgery at a week or so old. He had the successful life saving surgery on January 22, 2005. What happened to the DiMattio family cemented my commitment to the CMN runs.

Both of these runs would benefit Geisinger's Janet Weis Children's Hospital where Louis Carlo had his surgery. The first one was a 50-something mile run from JWCH in Danville, PA to the annual radiothon is Wilkes-Barre. I did not know the actual distance. I could only estimate it.

The second one would be a week long run from my adopted hometown of Covington Twp, PA to Philadelphia. I knew it was a 120-mile car ride and that I would have to take a more scenic route. I estimated the distance around 150 miles.

The training took a lot of time. More time on the road meant less time moping around the house. I got to think about Dad a lot. I came to a realization. He was a wonderful man with two horrible diseases. I was finally able, thanks to John Lemoncelli, to separate a great Dad from a bipolar alcoholic. When I thought about Dad, I always saw him in a more positive light than I used to. I would remember him quite fondly as I trained. I would dedicate these runs to two people. They would be in honor of Louis Carlo and in memory of Dad. When asked if I wanted to take two days to do the run I answered, "No that would not be a challenge."

I began my run at 8 a.m. at JWCH on a frigid February morning. I got on U.S. 11 which I would stay on for about 50 miles of the run. I came into the town of Bloomsburg and I saw a sign that said "Wilkes-Barre 38 miles." I knew at that moment that I would finish this run. Something told me that I easily had 38 miles left in my legs.

I was right. In about 10 hours (with breaks to eat) I finished the 56-mile (GPS measured) run. I wasn't even sore. I did this run on a Friday. On Sunday I ran a 10-miler with my eyes closed. I had come a long way from fighting for breath for ¼ mile at a 10-minute pace. Now it was time to set my sights on Philadelphia.

It was April 2005, and it was the day before The Boston Marathon was to be run. If you want the exact date, go look at a 2005 calendar. We had held a CMN carnival to raise money for the run. We raised 1,200 dollars that day and 800 more on my travels. I left the Covington Twp. fire department, where the carnival was held, and set my sights 30 miles away in Bartonsville. I was so full of adrenaline that I felt like I could fly there.

Thankfully, I was held in check by a good running buddy of mine named Jonathon Loiselle. I was capable of running that day in the 7:30s. He kept me in the 8:30-9-minute range. He saved my legs by setting me in that pace range. We ran the first 16 miles together. I would show up in Bartonsville 14 miles and 2 hours and 15 minutes later. I had picked up the pace to an 8-minute pace when left to my own devices. No matter though. My legs felt fine.

I spent the entire day on the road during the Monday that Boston was run. A documentary chronicling the run was being filmed, and the crew spent the better part of the day with me. There were a few running breaks due to the filming so when I stopped in Nazareth where I planned to stop for the night, I called my wife and told her to book me a hotel 10 miles away in Allentown.

It was sunset when I left Nazareth. I love running in the dark. I had a headlamp on and set out for Allentown. I cruised another 18 miles to a total of 43 for the day. I will not mention names, but there were people who were skeptical about my ability to do this run. When I got to Allentown in two days, I was serving up the crow topped with a nice cognac sauce.

Day 3 started early. I planned on sleeping until 10 a.m. You'd think I would be exhausted, but I wasn't. In fact, I felt refreshed. I was up by 6 and, after a fine free continental breakfast, was on the road by 9. I was headed toward Green Lane to the head of the Perkiomen Trail. It was 9 a.m., and it was already 75 degrees out. This was going to make for a long day.

I had about 20 miles in when I stopped for a Gatorade at a garage. They had a TV on. I walked in at the exact moment when Joseph Ratzenberger walked out onto the balcony as Pope Benedict XVI. Here I am, totally out of the loop, yet I saw a moment that I had been wondering about. Divine intervention strikes again. You think that was neat? Keep reading.

It was high noon and, as my buddy Jack Smedley puts it, hotter than the hammers of Hell. It was the first heat wave of 2005. It had to be at least 90 degrees out. The heat was rising off of the asphalt and, due to a traffic accident on the PA Turnpike, the traffic was rerouted to the road where I was running. I swear that the road was nothing but tractor trailers spewing black diesel exhaust into my air. The air quality was simply awful.

It was the afternoon, I had about 23 miles in, and I was starved. I found a TGI Friday's and ordered a Vanilla coke, breadsticks and chicken soup. I wanted to keep it bland.

I drank two cokes before the food showed up. It was a good thing, because, except for one breadstick and three spoonfuls of soup, it was all I could get into my stomach. "Oh great—my digestive system is shutting down." Since I couldn't eat, I stopped at a gas station, grabbed all the Gatorade my backpack could carry and got back on the road. I would have to subsist on gels and Gatorade. It was all I could tolerate.

I need to tell you some back story. Dad was in the Air Force. He was always looking above the horizon to point out contrails, the white cloudlike exhaust produced from a jet engine, in the sky. "Look at the contrail, Jay." He would point them out to me when I was a kid, and, when he got sick, would point them out to me when we took him outside.

We now return to our original programming already in progress.

It was around 2 p.m. It was 20 degrees warmer than it had any business being. I was hitting the wall so hard that I was walking any steep incline. I was on Route 663. It should have been Route 666, because I was in my own personal Hell. I was slamming down Gatorade, but it felt like I had a block of salt in my mouth. I was in the middle of nowhere, and the people I shared the apple with were at least 100 miles away. So I thought about whom we shared the apple for. I cried out loud.

"Lord? Dad? Anyone? If there was a time in my life when I needed your help, it is now."

I looked up. There it was—a jet plane flying right over my head, laying a contrail from where I had come to where I was headed. Coincidence? Definitely not. It was a sign from Heaven itself. I knew at that point that it would not get easier but I knew that I would get to Green Lane unscathed. I did just that. My friend—who am I kidding? I love him like a brother—Art Aubert was waiting for me.

I met Art at the expo of the 2003 Steamtown Marathon. I will talk to anybody anywhere. A friend of mine told me that I would talk to the corpse at a funeral. He's right. I talked to Dad a few times at the wake. Anyway, I had about a gallon of Gatorade resting on my bladder and had to let some of it go. I walked into the stall and there was a guy already in midstream.

"Dude, I've been going all day," he said.

"Tell me about it. But keep drinking; it's going to be hot tomorrow."

We gabbed a little more, then we went our separate ways. I thought nothing of it.

I needed to pack in some carbs (and let the inner fatman run amok), so I headed to Perkin's for my traditional five pancakes, five pieces of French toast, and a vanilla milkshake. Apparently, half the marathon had the same idea, because the place was packed. I gave my name for a table.

Who comes walking into the restaurant but the guy from one stall over. He was giving his name for a table. I walked over to him, "Look, I already gave my name. Why don't we eat together and talk about the race?"

"OK, sounds good. Art Aubert."

"Jay Sochoka."

That was the start of a great friendship. We exchanged e-mails and promised to connect after the Philadelphia Marathon, which we were both set to run. We did. We met before the race and then after it. He invited me to his post-race party. I accepted. We downed a few pints of lagered liquid carbohydrates together. It's very important to replace what you have lost after all. (Heh, heh).

We had stayed in touch by calls and e-mail. When it came time to do the Run to Philly, he did two things. He picked me up on Tuesday and took me to his house to crash until Thursday morning, and he volunteered to run with me on Thursday. We were figuring on covering 30 miles, leaving 10 for me on the last day so the documentary crew could film it.

It was Tuesday night, and we were hanging out in his hot tub, which I practically lived in from the moment I got there. We were having a beer (or six). "I want to run the last 40 miles with you. You want to put this thing to bed Thursday?" Art asked.

I thought about it. It was tempting to be done a day early. "Yeah. Let's do it!"

I had planned, à la Rocky, to finish on top of the first landing of the Philadelphia Museum of Art. I didn't want to spoil the ending, so I said, "I'll stop one step short of the landing."

"Don't worry about it," Art interjected "I don't want to run the steps anyway."

"OK. Done deal."

The next day Art and I ran an errand. We wanted to do something special during this run. There was a war going on, after all. We bought the biggest flag we could comfortably carry and run at the same time. We would change it two miles at a time. It would be a tribute to all of the soldiers past and present, living and dead.

Thursday morning arrived, and we were driven to the Perkiomen Trailhead where I had finished on Tuesday. We would run on it for 20 miles then we would get on the Canal Path for the last 20. We started out flying. The first 10 miles and five flag handoffs flew right by. I was feeling good, and Art looked great. I knew he was going to do it. We took a camera with us to chronicle the feat.

We were cruising right along when at mile 30 my phone rang. It was home calling.

"Hello?"

"Jesse's dead," Sheryl sobbed. "She got hit by a car."

I don't remember the conversation after that. I just remember how awful I felt. With Dad gone, Jesse was all that my Mom had. Looking back, we noticed that Jesse was never the same after Dad died. She was at his side now, where she belonged. I got off the phone and kept running. I had job to do.

We passed a sign that said "Welcome to Philadelphia" on the Canal Path Trail. Art was laboring now. He was concentrating so hard that he didn't even see the sign. I felt fine, but this was going to be a fight for Art. "OK, Art, we'll run your pace now." I stayed by his side the whole time.

We got into the Mannyunk part of Philadelphia. We were six miles from finishing. "I need to grab a Coke," Art said. We found a bar and took a break.

"Where are you running from?" the bartender asked.

"He came from Scranton, I started in Green Lane."

You could hear the clang as the bartenders jaw hit the floor. We finished our drinks and set out for the finish. We were about two miles out.

"Jay?"

"Yeah Art?"

"I'm going to run the steps!"

"Give me the camera, Art."

We pounded the steps, and I stopped one short. He went to the landing and we celebrated Art's first 40-mile run. We celebrated further after we hobbled to South

Street for burgers and beer. We truly felt like Masters of the Universe.

The next day the film crew caught up with me. I reran the last two miles of the run as they filmed it. In total, I would run 156 miles in 4½ days. I made it to the landing where they had people gathered for the finish. They actually had a finish line tape set up for me. I never broke a tape before. I roared a victory cry after I broke the tape. Braveheart did not scream as long or as loud. Another pure victory.

That run was cathartic. It helped me put a lot in perspective. It showed me that I had a power greater than myself looking out for me. Do I believe in an afterlife? No doubt. Here's why.

Sometime after that run, I had a dream. I was at the lake standing at the end of the dock. It was an overcast, yet hot and humid day. I could actually feel the warmth and humidity. It was a perfect day to spend lakeside. My favorite kind of lake day. Dad's too. I shouldn't have been surprised when he showed up.

He was wearing his trademark brown bathing suit and was about 50 years old. He was completely restored. "I just want you to know I'm okay," he said. "I like it here."

He didn't mean Newton Lake; he meant Heaven. This was not a dream, it was a vision. I was with Dad in Heaven. I guess Heaven does look a lot like Newton Lake. I told him that I was happy for him, I missed him, and I loved him.

"I love you too. I have to go now. You can't come with me yet. I just want to let you know I'm all right."

He then got into a boat. Not the Mastercraft ski boat that he bought me, but our first boat. His boat. "I always knew you liked that one better." The engine started, the boat pulled away, and he was gone. I awoke from the vision awash with peace.

I called Mom first thing the next morning and told her what happened. It gave her a lot of comfort to know that Dad was okay.

It has been five and a half years, at the time of this writing, since Dad died. Life has rolled on. I have had my ups and had my downs. Julian has gone from a toddler to a nine-year old boy. He still remembers his Pop-Pop. It comforts me to know that. I think about him everyday. How could I not?

15

It's Not About the Clock

St. George: "I'm bringing you in on a 4-12."
The Dragon:"A 4-12? WHAT'S A 4-12?!"
St. George: "Overacting."
—From Stan Freeberg's "St. George and the Dragon Net"

Y OU might be wondering what the above quote has to do with running.

The answer is nothing and everything. I associate it with the 2005 Steamtown Marathon, because it is from a Stan Freeberg bit that used to crack Dad up. Mom was not a big fan of the album (yes, it was a vinyl LP)~just not her type of comedy. It wasn't dirty; it just didn't tickle her funny bone. It would, however, put Dad and me in stitches every time we listened to it. I actually have the boxed set of Stan Freeberg's works on CD and listen to it from time to time; satirical comedy at its finest. So, to answer the question, that quote had to do with Dad, which had everything to do with my Steamtown Marathon weekend from the expo to the race.

Chris Kelly's article moved me to tears, and I was there for the interview. That's how good a writer he is. You may want to reach for the Kleenex. Here it is.

October 8, 2005

26 miles is nothing when a man is running for his life

Jay Sochoka keeps a fat man in his pocket and a dead man in his heart.

When the miles rise like mountains and his will fades in valley shadow, they carry him home.

"I think of him every time I lace up my shoes," Jay says of his dad, Joe, who died in January.

"I carry a picture of him wherever I go," he says of the fat man, who hasn't been seen in the flesh for years but is very much alive inside Jay's athletic, 198-pound frame.

There was a time when Jay would have howled at the notion of his name and "athletic" sharing space in a sentence.

He says his dad would have joined him.

That was before Jay traded two daily packs of Marlboro Lights for a tin of "curiously strong" peppermints. Before he walked away from McDonald's and into Weight Watchers. Before he passed the elevator on his way to the treadmill. Before he converted the garage of his Moscow home into a gym.

Before he started running for his life.

"I'm not skinny," he says, using an index finger for punctuation.

"I'm a fat man in recovery. I've been food sober for five years."

Five years ago, Jay weighed 306 pounds. At 29, he had 15 years of on-and-off Weight Watchers membership under his belt. He had graduated from husky to big-and-tall, and was working on a master's degree in unhealthy living.

He and Sheryl had been married four years, and were thinking about starting a family.

"I said to myself, 'Man, I want to be able to run and play with my kids," he says. "I don't want to be the kind of dad who just sits around on the couch all the time."

So he got off the couch and into a gym. He watched what he ate. He walked to work and around Lake Scranton. When walking became too easy, he ran. And ran. And ran.

On Sunday, Jay will run his fifth Steamtown Marathon, striving for a finish time that qualifies him for the Boston Marathon, a goal he missed by a mere 40 seconds last year.

If not for a minute-long "pit-stop" at the 9-mile mark, Jay says he'd already be booked for Beantown.

This year's race, the marathon's 10th edition, will be bittersweet for Jay no matter how well he runs. Sheryl, their son Julian, 4, and Jay's mother, Judy, will be cheering at Mulberry Street and Washington Avenue, near the race's downtown Scranton finish.

Joe Sochoka won't.

"I can trace Dad's disease in the four years he saw me run," Jay says. "From the first, where he stood at the corner of Mulberry and Washington and cheered with a 'That's my son' look on his face to last year's, when he was wheelchair-bound and we pretty much knew it was the last race he would see me run.

"I remember coming over that last hump at Mulberry and I screamed to him, 'I love you!' at the top of my lungs. He called that night and told me how proud he was. I thanked him for coming out to cheer me on. There was a silence and then I heard a sniffle. I knew he was crying. I was, too."

Tears come easy as Jay looks back on the last years of his dad's life. He had multiple system atrophy, a rare and always fatal neurological disorder that methodically shuts down its victims like an engineer preparing a condemned building for demolition.

Watching his dad waste away was doubly frustrating for Jay. A pharmacist, he spent his days dispensing thousands of medications for everything from high blood pressure to sexual enhancement while knowing that nothing on the shelf would put his dad back on his feet.

Some nights, he'd stay with his dad so Mom could take a break. He'd carry him to the bathroom. He'd carry him to the kitchen.

He'd carry him.

As his dad's life ebbed, Jay found solace in running. He logs about 50 to 60 miles a week, 70 to 80 when he's gearing up for a race.

He's run several marathons, but he's most at home on Steamtown's winding grind from Forest City to Scranton.

"I know every corner of that road," he says, adding that many spectators know him by his signature American flag running shirt. "The people are just great and the cheering means so much when you're out there. If there's a home-field advantage, I've got it."

And Jay says everyone has what it takes to make the kinds of changes that got him off the sidelines and into the race. He'll be sharing tips on "Finding the Runner in Me" today at 1 p.m. at the Race Expo at Scranton High School.

"Anyone has the power within to do what I did," he says. "The key is to harness it and use it correctly. The process is a marathon, not a sprint. Slow and steady wins the race. To finish is to win."

Jay's running shirt carries a tribute to his father and the day his race ended. Jay says it's a way to have his dad with him when he reaches Mulberry and Washington.

"I wouldn't be surprised if I saw him there, just for a second," Jay says. "He'll be with me in spirit. Hopefully, during parts of the race when it gets tough, he can help carry me home."

If you're out watching the race tomorrow and you see a red, white and blue running shirt with "DAD 1-22-05" printed on the back, that's Joe Sochoka's son rising from the valley, conquering the mountains, shredding the shadows.

Cheer him on. Wave him forward. Carry him home.

CHRIS KELLY, Times-Tribune columnist,
E-mail: kellysworld@timesshamrock.com

Good, you're back. Now on with the show.

The booth at the expo was a success. I talked to so many runners and took countless blood pressures and blood glucose readings. Not to mention the 18 cases of Gatorade I gave away. Give Gatorade, and they will come.

"The Never Ending Road," went very well. It ran longer than I had planned, because I was ad-libbing a bit. I was more comfortable with the material this year, so I was able to run off of the pages a bit. I actually would up cutting material out just so the next presentation could go on. People came up to me later and said how inspired they were. I had done my job.

My right foot was sore all day, so I was a bit worried about the race. I admit to you now that I was more injured than I let on.

After the expo, we parked my car by the finish and went to the runners' Mass at the expo. Father, and runner, Jeff

Walsh officiated the service. He read a passage from Dr. George Sheehan talking about how becoming a runner becomes so intertwined in our beings that it defines who we are. That is why, even though injured, I had to run this race. I am a runner. It's what I do.

After Mass, Sheryl and I went to "Irene the Machine's" house (Irene Cobb is a phenomenal local Master's runner) for a pasta dinner with the Keystone group. We were halfway there when all of a sudden I let out a long stream of profanity.

After my wife asked what was wrong, I told her that my bib and chip were in my truck in the parking deck. Between the all-day rain, my sore foot, and now this, I seemed to have a full-blown disaster on my hands. Everything was telling me not to run. My wife has a slightly better perspective. "Better to remember you forgot your bib now than at 4 a.m." Good point, dear.

We had a good time at the dinner. We were all a bit revved up, but tried to stay as low-key as possible. It was great to be with my best running friends the night before such an important race. Ned Clarke was coming back from a layoff, Nancy Werthmuller was running her 10th Steamtown, Irene was shooting for a PR, Paul Fahey and Mike Kozlansky were making their debuts, Vicki was shooting for a 3:10, and Jonathan was looking to run a BQ 3:15.59 on the chip. I was sticking to my "3:10 as long as the foot holds" story.

After the party, Sheryl and I went to Mom's house to get some sleep. She lives five miles from the start so it makes sense to stay there before the race. I sandwiched my foot between two Lidoderm patches and put it in the night splint. I fell right to sleep and got a full six hours. Not bad for the night before a race.

I got up, had my Rice Krispies with milk, took my medications, and had a cup of coffee. After Sheryl came downstairs, we headed out to Forest City. The foot felt great. If it could hold up, I could qualify for Boston. Amazingly enough, the rain had stopped, except for a fine mist, and there was a tailwind. Absolutely perfect weather for a marathon.

When I arrived at Forest City, I was the first runner there. I took a warm-up and the foot felt fine. If it could hold up for 26 miles, I would be OK. In the hours before the race, I pretty much saw all of my running buddies. All of them said I had 3:10 in the bag. Having more detailed knowledge of my condition, I was skeptical. I put on my arch brace and put two rounds of tape around it. It felt well-supported.

Walking onto the starting grid, I started to feel the pre-race vibe—1,800 runners were filled with excitement. The field was blessed, the national anthem was sung, and the Civil War brigade fired the cannon. Well they almost fired the cannon. The gunpowder was wet and we were started with a pistol. A minute or so later, the cannon went off, scaring me and the rest of the field.

Church bells rang us out of Forest City in honor of Steamtown's 10th anniversary, and I hit the first mile split in 7:42. Not bad, considering the time to the mat and the traffic. I moved past Irene and Nancy and up to Mike. If I could run with him again (We had a practice 20-miler a month earlier), we would be set. We hit mile 2 in 7:21, which set us up nicely for the big downhill. My foot started to twinge here and there, but it was not bad.

The Mile 3 split came and the news was not good. 7:48 and the more downhill the course became, the more pain

I was in. I knew at that point that it was not about Boston. Mere survival was at hand on this course. Since I no longer cared about mile splits, I will not announce every mile. I did log them out of habit.

On the way down to Carbondale, Ned, Irene, and Nancy went by me. They were concerned for me. I told them not to worry. I would hang with them for as long as I could. I did not hang on that long, and they were going down the hill. They looked great.

Father Walsh came upon me next. Once again, my steps lightened. Talking with him about my father and Our Father, we ran a decent pace. Also, I volunteered to play guitar at next year's Mass. He thought that it was a great idea. He went on, and I was on my own again.

I talked to runners here and there and had fun with the fans who, despite the weather, came out in force to cheer us on. My foot hurt with every stride. I began to think of Dad and how his abilities left him. I also thought how he never quit. Up until the very end, he tried to live life as independently as he could. I would not quit. If I had to walk to a six-hour marathon, I would. There would be no getting me off the course.

We hit Carbondale, and were greeted by the fans, band, and cheerleaders. They seemed especially rowdy. I was way off the clock, but I was having a blast. I was worried about my foot, which didn't hurt as much as long as I didn't push it. I was also worried about my wife. What would she think when I did not hit Archbald by 9:40?

On the way to Mayfield, I passed Nancy. Her foot gave out, also. She said she'd finish, no matter how long it took. That inspired me a bit more. I was not alone in my situation. I ran with Bill Lawrence a bit after that. He is always a riot to talk to. He was having issues in the bushes having to stop quite frequently. He knows I'm a pharmacist and asked if I had any saw palmetto on me. The laughing took the concentration off of my foot.

We cruised through Mayfield, and I heard people shouting for me. People I did not even know. Apparently, a lot of people read Chris Kelly. They were indeed helping to carry me home.

As the race went on, people would pass me or I would pass them and they would say, "You really inspired me yesterday. That was such a great story." It made me feel good that I did my job. It wasn't really a job. It was just the story of my running life.

I got to Archbald and saw my wife, Mom, and Julian in the distance. Julian was jumping and cheering for me. He had grown so much. Five Steamtowns earlier, he was sleeping in a stroller. I pulled off the course and gave him a big kiss and hug. I took a Red Bull from Sheryl and told her, "Don't worry about mile 23, just go to the finish."

I got back on the course and hit the trail. The Red Bull kicked in and I felt good on the trails. They were also in great shape. They were soft on top but solid on the bottom. I feel like I did not lose any time on them. It was also quite beautiful. "Run with the water," I said to myself.

We hit Jessup, and the fans were indeed wild, lining the trail on both sides. High -fiving and shouting all the way. I heard out of the corner of my ear, "Run, son." I didn't see who said it and there was no one around me. Maybe that was the "For a second" I talked about in the article. It was around mile 17, and I thought about crossing Washington and Mulberry. Instantly my eyes watered up. "Save it for when you get there," I said to myself and pressed on.

At the 21 split, I saw a man walking. It was Father Walsh, reduced to a walk and a hurt one at that.

"Father," I said.

"Pray for me," was his reply.

As I rounded the corner, I broke into tears. It hurt to see him hurting. Just like it hurt to see Dad fail. "Come on, we still have five miles to go," I said to myself, sucked it up and kept moving.

At mile 23, Ned Clarke was walking up the first nasty hill in the set. As I went by him he shouted an, "I'm with you, brother."

"And I'm with you," I replied and marched on. Part of me wanted to walk with him, but the other part wanted to get off of this course as soon as possible. I glanced at my watch and it looked like I would break 3:40. I felt pretty good about that.

I raced across Boulevard Avenue and looked at Electric Street. There was the hill. I spit on it as I started up. I would not walk a step today. I may not be running my fastest, but I would not walk. I made my way up and the crowds were crazy.

At the top of Electric Street, I did something that I never did at the race.

I'm usually on the clock and cut the corner short, but this time I took a few seconds and went up to the children and gave high-fives and shook hands with those who could. Two miles from the finish, and I started crying again. Sometimes it's not about the clock.

Down the hill on Sunset Avenue and around and onto Capouse, I started to cruise. I gave whatever sprint my foot would give me. I hit 25 and made the last turn onto Washington Avenue. I looked at the hill and laughed. I would climb it, and the corner would be waiting for me. I made it right up to Cooper's without a problem. Before I hit the Masonic Temple, I passed a young woman and said, "We're Home." She smiled and I went on my way.

Over the top, I got to the corner of Washington and Mulberry. I went flying down the hill and headed for the finish line. The crowd was packed and people were screaming. At 3:35 flat, I crossed the line pointing to the heavens, closing a chapter in the book of my life. There will be other Steamtown marathons without my Dad, but that was the first.

I was reunited with my family, and we all laughed and cried a little. Dad 1/22/05 on my singlet said it all.

I did not run a PR. I finished a nothing happens by accident 412 and ran a P-U as far as my abilities are concerned. I ran the best race I could that day, and sometimes, that has to be enough.

To finish is to win. Always.

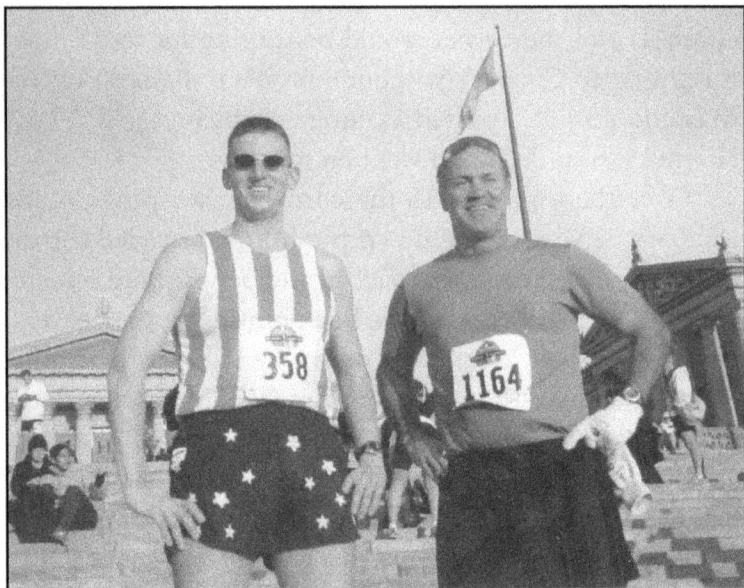

Jay and Art at the Philadelphi Museum of Art at the 2003 Philadelphia Marathon (Yes, they named the museum after Art.)

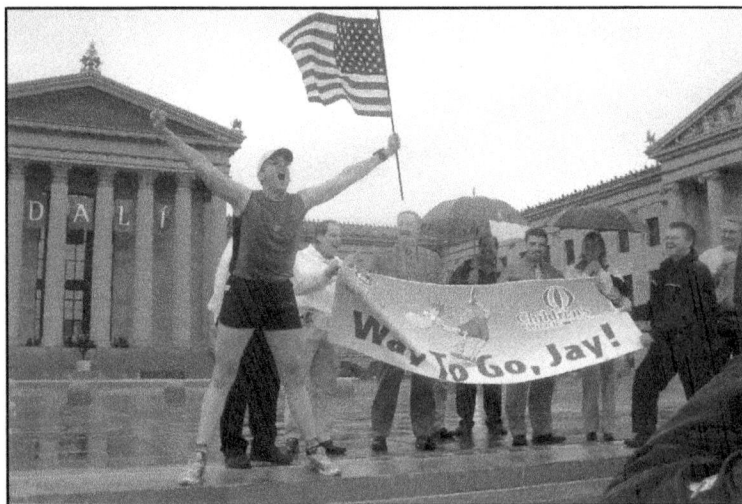

156 miles in 5 days to benefit Children's Miracle Network

16

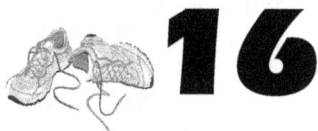

The Road to Boston Goes Through Scranton
Part I

Author's Note: The following three chapters contain some mild potty humor. There are two reasons for this. 1) It is highly relevant to the story. 2) When you have to take care of a loved one's bathroom needs, you get desensitized. 3) Potty humor is hysterical. Let's face it. Everybody poops, and runners poop in some pretty strange places. I dare you to show me a single runner who has not gone "al fresco." If you are not a fan of Mel Brooks, and therefore easily offended, look out for the brackets, [ ], and scan past those passages.

October 8, 2006 4:45 a.m. Race Day

With the alarm set for 5 a.m., I shut it off and leapt out of bed.

I took a shower and had a very light breakfast. I was pretty full from the previous night. I ate Italian food at a local restaurant. My wife thought the Bolognese sauce tasted burnt; she refused to eat it and warned me to not eat too much. I ate three bowlfuls and thought nothing of it. That day, I had a small bowl of Cookie Crisp with a little milk and a cup of coffee. After the coffee hit, I felt the need for my morning elimination.

[Usually I don't discuss this, but trust me on this one. It was a dandy. Usually, I struggle to pass a green bean. This was more like a banana with the monkey's arm still attached to it. I said to myself (since no one else was up), "Wow. No need to even bring paper towels with me." I took it along just in case. Usually when I bring it, I never need it. If I forget it, I'm reaching for leaves.]

I went upstairs, prepped my feet with Aquaphor and blister powder, and got dressed. I looked at the back of my singlet. "DAD" and "UNK" would be carried with me. "UNK" was for my Uncle Mike, who had sadly passed away two months prior to race day. I put on my signature navy and star shorts (half of my "Unfaded Glory" outfit) and prepared to get my game face on. I still had socks to choose. Usually, I wear my American Flag socks, but, since I had new top, I had to go with new socks. Well, one anyway. I put on a "Flash" logo sock with a flag sock.

I am part superhero on race day after all.

I grabbed my Garmin and got in my car. For the first time, I would take the bus from Scranton to the starting line in Forest City. As I was driving down, I was blasting my stereo and listening to some aggressive hardcore metal. It got me really ready to go. I parked my car in the deck, and while it was pitch black out, put on my sunglasses.

To paraphrase the Blues Brothers, "We've got a full belt of gels, and half a bottle of Gatorade. It's dark out, and we're wearing sunglasses. Hit it!" The race was two hours away, but it was already show time.

I took the scenic route to the mall where the buses were. I took a look at the finish line. *I'll see you in about 5 hours and 15 minutes.* It was 6 a.m. Do the math. I then moved on.

"If there's anything more important than my ego around, I want it caught and shot now." –Zaphod Beeblebrox
From *The Hitchhiker's Guide to the Galaxy*, Chapter 12, by Douglas Adams

It is time. Time to transform. From Clark Kent to Superman. From Gene Simmons abused parent and un-husband (check out Gene Simmons' Family Jewels) to "The Demon." Rock and Roll's Dark Lord of bass. From Jay Sochoka, former 300-pounder and mild-mannered pharmacist (Actually, mild-mannered might be a stretch!), to Captain America (Lackawanna Trail High School's nickname for me), an Iron Horse marathon runner, who will finish with a select few heavyweights dispersed with the running twigs.

I am a superhero. I am Rock and Roll. I am going to attempt to qualify for Boston for I run with power and strength. I may not be 150 pounds, but that does not matter. For my size, I AM SPEED!

As I walked to the bus local runners, Jim Moran, Spike Lynott, and John Major all wished me luck. "See you in about three hours," Spike said as I hopped on. I just smiled and nodded. I was feeling it today.

"GOOD MORNING, LADIES!" I said in my best R. Lee Ermy voice. Everyone looked at me like I was certifiable. I am. It was appropriate that I was wearing my Bubba Gump Shrimp Co. hat, because no one was offering me a spot on the bus. I wonder why?

"You can sit here." It wasn't Jenny, but it was a familiar face. I met Mark Cox at the CMN Carnival 5K. He is powerfully built and is destined to be an ultra runner. We talked about a lot of things, but the one was doing the CMN radiothon ultra together and adding about 15 miles to it. We would start at the school where he teaches. He had the kids working the math for his race. The good old "RTD" problem: rate, time, and distance. They were calculating his pace, total time, mile splits—you name it. Totally awesome concept.

After messing with a rookie's mind for a bit, we were at Forest City H.S. and got off the bus. For those who have not run Steamtown, you have to see it to believe it. Volunteer students are all over the place: directing, leading, handing out water, and whatever else needs to be done. But wait, that's not all. The Cheerleading Squad is there and full of pep. As we got off the bus, the cheerleaders were whooping it up for us.

I gave some back. "HELLO, FOREST CITYYYYYY!" I said in my best Paul Stanley meets Steven Tyler. I am Rock and Roll after all.

After being led to the big gym and parting ways with Mark and his crew, I went to the cafeteria. I was not hungry, but this is where the pace groups set up. I threw my bag under the Sub-3:10 sign and set out for the facilities (aka The Head, John, Hopper, etc). The indoor plumbing usually open until 7 a.m. [Since everything was ok with "The Deuce" department, I just needed to drain a few gallons from my bladder. I did not want to have to stop for that again and have it cost me Boston. I stood in line. After a few minutes of waiting, I realized there was no flushing going on. I looked around the corner, and the stand-ups were wide open.

There's a definite need for some line signage on the outer men's room—one for the Thrones and one for the Stand-ups. "#1's" and "2's" would get the point across pretty delicately and save the male runners some severe nasal passage trauma. I don't know what we all eat, but wow! (I could drop another line in here but I don't want to offend...yet).]

I went back into the café and talked to a Master's Runner named Jeff. He was from Florida. Flat and warm Florida.

"So, you came up here to run up and down hills and freeze to death." He replied in the affirmative and also indicated that this was his first Steamtown. "Run the first half easy and don't try to bank time on the first long downhill after two (miles)," which, in one form or another, is my traditional rookie advice. I was talking to Jeff when he walked in.

"BOB!"

Bob Lutzick and I made our marathon debut together at Steamtown in 2001. We were so nervous/excited that we kept talking each other down. We shared the goal of finishing, but our timeframes differed slightly. We lined up together, but we knew we would not stay together long. He finished and I finished. As bad as I am with names (I apologize for this), I always remember Bob. I have used "Bro," "Man," "Brother," "Bud," any other informal nickname on people for as long as three years until I finally picked up on someone's name in a conversation. It is an awful flaw and, again, I apologize. I only knew Bob as Bob. I just learned his last name that race day.

The local 3:10 group started to show up. This is the once a year group of comedians, off-color jokesters, and not very slow runners.

It is one laugh after another. We really keep each other loose. Billy Cadden (stocky statistical anomaly), Kevin

Bandru (pace master extraordinaire), Scranton Fire Chief Tommy Davis (ageless wonder), Mark Fueshko, Ed "The Hammer" Gavin, Jim Walsh, and the rest of the court jesters (myself included) were in form.

After warming up the sense of humor, I took a brisk one-mile run—just enough to get the legs going. The cheerleaders were cheering as I went by, cross country team members gave me the "Rock & Roll" sign (pinky and index finger up middle, ring, down thumb tucked in) after I flashed it to them. I did some high fives and started to wrap it up. Until he tapped me on the shoulder.

Mike Kozlansky sidled next to me, and I went about ¼ mile further. We both felt great and ready to really do something out there.

Mike is a tremendous tri-athlete and a very gifted runner. During a 23-mile training run, I had to work just to keep up with him. At the end of it, he went into a sprint. I just watched him go. He was amazing. Had it not been for my foot the previous year, we would have been together for a while. He also weighs 208 pounds and is not going to get any smaller. I was in the Iron Horse division as well, but I had him picked to win it. More on him in another passage.

Dave Kennedy finally showed up. Since he was the youngest of the group he actually needed a 3:10 to qualify for Boston. For the rest of us, it was just a personal goal. Dave was as wound up as I was. I told him we would huddle up before the race started.

We went back to the pace group area and made our final preparations. I wrote a large "J" on each shoulder with a marker. It was enough of my name to get the point across.

We headed out to the back of the school to use the "outdoor plumbing" one last time. As we were walking toward the start, time seemed to stand still, and everything seemed to move in slow motion. The WNEP-16 helicopter was warming up for takeoff, and so were we. I wished runners good luck and gave the nervous ones a nod of encouragement. Showtime was 10 minutes away. As we gathered toward the seven-minute pace sign, Dave and I lost the pace group. We could not find a person we knew.

We huddled up and reminded ourselves to be patient, take it easy in the start, and not blow what we have worked all year for. We were about five minutes from finding out if all of our hard work paid off.

The national anthem was sung, the runners were blessed, and it was about time to get rolling. The hand cyclist took off and the runners were on deck.

The Civil War Brigade stood ready at the cannon. "Runner's ready...set..."

17

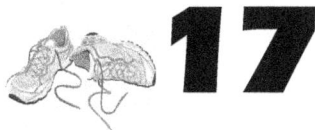

The Road to Boston Goes Through Scranton
Part II

BOOM!

A FTER the traditional startled rookie collective scream, we were off. The opening street is a bit narrow, so it is a little slow going to the line and for the first ¼ mile or so. I tend to "Moo" at this point. The cattle in the paddock reference usually gets a few laughs.

Dave and I set out to work through the crowd a bit. We broke apart but were within sight of each other. We were shouting to each other as we were moving through.

We were together by mile 1 at 7:18. That included 19 seconds to the start line. Not only was the pace dialed in, it was 15 seconds under where we had to be. Mile 2 was the same thing (6:52). This was through some slightly hilly terrain as well. The big glide does not start until mile 3 (6:54) which was an attempt by Dave and me to "slow down" from our sub 3-hour marathon pace. We were indeed running at "ludicrous speed." (Thank you, Mr. Mel Brooks).

Speed kills, but speed thrills, especially in this race. Dave and I were ripping on the long glide. We had caught up to Cads (Billy Cadden) and then proceeded to laugh our way through the next couple miles. Due to the adult nature of most of the jokes being cracked, they will not be mentioned here. Let it just be said that adrenaline is a hell of a drug. Miles 4, 5, & 6 went 7:01, 6:48, and 6:52 respectively. The 7:01 came from changing my watch to manual splits because I came in long on the first mile. After that, it all lined up.

Dave kept asking me if I was OK holding this pace. I told him that if I didn't want to run it this way, I'd drop back. I was in my comfort zone and holding my own no problem. I knew the chances of burning up on re-entry were good, but I figured that even if I hit the wall, I could keep going and take a 3:15 to Boston.

We ripped through Fell Twp., Simpson, and Upper Carbondale. The crowds and aid stations were phenomenal. There was even a live band back in Vandling around mile 3 on the course. It's 8:30 in the morning and people are on their porches clapping for us. I still cannot believe the support that this race draws from the towns. I guess since we are blocking the roads to church, we are the only show in town. Incidentally, mile 7 was a 6:58.

Speaking of a show in town, you have to run this race just to run through Carbondale. The rush of adrenaline is simply amazing. My skin tingles as I hear the marching band, the cheerleaders, and the frenzied crowd. It took all the holding back possible just to run a 6:48. Dave actually went faster that that. He had pulled ahead of me. I passed Chief Davis at this point.

"Hey Tommy," I said.

"Go get 'em ," he replied.

He appeared to be working harder than normal at this point. T.D. calls me his hero, which is funny, because he is one of mine. I think he's 60. He is still muscular and usually pops a 3:10-ish marathon.

I took Tommy's advice and caught up back to Dave. He had slowed a bit and mile 9 came in at a 6:58. We then got to talking again. I was catching my breath, so I let him start.

"My Dad will be giving me a hand-off under the bridge," he said. "When I first told him I was going to run a marathon he said there was no way I could do it. Now he's my biggest fan."

I told him I felt the same way and how I became in my Dad's eyes, "My son, the athlete," after finishing my first Steamtown.

I then remembered who I was running for.

God

Dad

Unk

Brent

You know the first three, but I'm sure you are asking, "Who is Brent?" He's not on the shirt. He may not be— neither is God, I might add—but he is in my heart with the other three.

Brent Letersky was my brother—my fraternity brother, to be exact, but my brother nonetheless. I was a bit of an anomaly in college. I was not the norm, but Brent hung out with me anyway. We always cracked each other up. We would watch the movie *Major League* and still laugh. Anytime I watch or quote that movie, which is quite often, I think of him. Other brothers came to my wedding; he drove the 250 or so miles from Mechanicsburg, PA, to Old Bridge, NJ, to come to my bachelor party. He was my brother indeed.

He was 30 years old when he died in August 2004. I was crushed when I heard the news from another brother,

Mark "Spin" Gartner. The last time I saw him was my wedding. I always meant to call and never did. At the memorial service, there was a painting and his ashes. I was ok with that. I was really nervous about seeing his body. Whether it was Brent's wishes or the family's, I'm glad I was spared the trauma. He will be forever missed by me. God bless you, Brent "Squirrel" Letersky, R.Ph. Watch over us.

Dave took the handoff and we hit 10 in 6:51. "Do you think we should slow down?" Dave asked. "Can you?" I retorted.

We just kept running. Caution to the wind and "Flirting with Disaster" (Molly Hatchett—Google the song if you do not know it. Listen to it, then drop me an e-mail telling me how it applies to the marathon). We just kept ripping up the road and drove towards not only Boston, but a wicked PR. Mayfield and Jermyn (especially by the Windsor Inn) are very well supported. Local runners go to different vantage points. Carbondale and Jermyn are two of them.

We clicked by 11 at 6:59. We almost hit 7, and I was out of my comfort zone. My stomach also bothered me a bit. I remembered my wife's words of caution. That burnt sauce felt like it was coming back to haunt me. I thought that there was no possible way, since my high colonic at 5 a.m. We caught up to Cads, and he said to us, "Meat on the bone boys. Meat on the bone." The only problem with that is when you cut off the meat, you sometimes hit the bone.

Mile 12 was a 7:08. "DAMN!" We were starting to lose it. I knew it. I would make Boston, probably, but a 3:10 was going to be a fight. Bring it on, I thought to myself. I tried to take a gel (chocolate) but half of it exploded in my hand.

Mile 13 was a 7:07 with a total time of 1:30:43 we hit the 13.1 at 1:31 something. I didn't split it because I wanted to keep my miles intact. This was my fastest half ever in a marathon by at least two minutes, maybe three. With my rate of decline I was using the multiply by 2 and add 10 minute method to the time. I was projecting a 3:13, but I could probably better that. I scared myself, because I did the math wrong and came up with 3:23. I added 20 by mistake.

It did, however, get me moving—in more ways than one.

[Past the half there were three port-a-johns. Dave, who had pulled slightly ahead of me, ran in one. I could either pass him or jump in the open one. It looked like a slot machine that hit 3 cherries. I was in the women's one, but any port in the storm. I was quick, but because my hands were so sweaty, and coated in chocolate gel, the paper was sticking to my hand. I was pitching an out loud fit. I heard laughing as Cads went by. Dave left, and I followed him after I got my hand cleaned off. I had to or no one in their right mind would have handed me a Gatorade or water the way it was.

Toilet paper and brown colored gel. Would you hand me water?]

This caused me to hit mile 14 in 7:54. Still sub-8. "Impressive," I thought to myself. Notice I said myself. I had let Dave go on. I had to keep running my own race. That required me to slow down.

My wife was about a quarter mile up the road with a Red Bull. I needed it. I took the drink and threw her my horribly fogged up sunglasses. They were in my back pocket since mile 4. Marathons are dangerous when you can't see.

"You look great!" she said.

It is better to look good than feel good, I thought to myself. I felt crappy. Literally. [I drank my Red Bull, hit the first trail section and proceeded to fart so badly that the leaves were falling off the trees]. Mile 15 came on the trail at 7:15. Just over 3:10 pace, but I had some time in the bank. It was a ton of work to keep that pace on the trails. Mile 16 came in at 7:24. I was getting sapped and could be facing a full meltdown.

Mile 17 was a 7:20. The crowds on the sides of the trails pushed me. This section in Peckville is a great crowd spot. They give you just enough room to run but you can reach out and high five them. It is totally awesome.

[I finally stopped farting somewhere around here—much to the relief of those behind me. I generated many a "Man! Are you OK?!"]

We then hit town again (Jessup, I believe), and I saw cousin Bill. He cheered me on. We then entered Mellow Park. 7:33 was the split. "Oh Boy, here we go." I was getting worried. I could not do the math to realize I had 1 hour and 15 minutes to run 8.2 miles for a BQ (runner speak for a Boston Qualifying time).

We looped around Mellow Park and onto the Wood-chip trail to Condella Park. We came over the bridge and there they were. "MARYWOOD!" I screamed. My homies, the Marywood Cross-Country team, went ballistic.

The coach and I recognize each other by face not name. "C'mon, Big Guy! Looking great!" he said. I suppose I looked okay. I hit 19 in 7:40. I was glad to get off the woodchips. Nothing now but road from here to Downtown Scranton.

I was giving all now. I hit 20 with an 8:02. I was starting to panic. Kyle Kozlansky (Mike's son) ran out to give me another Red Bull. "Where's your Dad?!" I asked. I had not seen him all race. I thought that I could have been in front of him.

"He's a few minutes ahead of you. Go get him!" he replied. So much for wishful thinking. I legged out a 7:06 to 21. "Okay, Okay. That's more like it. C'mon baby," I was thinking out loud. My stomach was too quirky to take gels, so I left them in my pockets. No big deal. I'd be fine. On the way to 22 the sub 3:10 group passed me. We were in front of them the whole time. "C'mon, 3:10!" Kevin Bandru said.

"I need a 3:15, and I'm pretty spent up. Go ahead."

"3:15...You got it! Keep it up!" Kevin kept going with Paul O'Hora and Marty Noll in tow. Mile 22 rolled in at a 7:36.

Mile 23 was an 8:10. Here's why.

[Round Two of the gastric battle was rearing its ugly head. I found a grassy clearing that was semi-secluded, dropped trow as discreetly as possible (only the back end showed) and let it rip. The blast pattern resembled that of a Claymore mine. I finished up, much to the snickering of a few runners, and got moving.

On the other side of the bridge was a pristine unused port-o-pot. I laughed myself into hysterics.]

When I came across 23, I looked at my total time. 2:46:50. 5K = 3.1 miles in 28 minutes. I was going.

I knew I had done it and felt the rush. It helped move me up that first hill to the Convenient Mart. It got me ripping across Boulevard Ave. It did not, however carry me all the way up Electric Street. I came to the bottom of the hill and was laboring.

A couple was at the bottom looking in the paper to match my name to my bib number. I frantically and breathlessly pointed to my shoulder. "C'mon Jay! Almost home!" they shouted.

I tried to run the entire hill—I did—but I had to walk a bit. I was wasting too much energy. I power walked it with most of the runners around me. "When in Rome," I thought.

That was until Vince Fedor (local runner and coach) jumped into the course and with both hands motioned me forward like he was pulling me. "C'MON!" he screamed. I ran toward and past him. Tim Welby (local pediatrician and marathon fanatic) cheered me up the rest of the hill. The kids from St. Joseph's were there. I had time, so I gave them High fives. Mile 24 clocked in at an 8:13.

I came down the hill and got my legs back under me. I ran by a woman walking. "C'mon, run with me. We're almost home. We're going to Boston," I said calmly. She nodded and started up. We are all teammates out there.

I ran a 7:48 into 25. I saw Faith Loiselle doing traffic, "I'm Frakking Going to Boston!" I excitedly whispered to her. She cracked up laughing.

"ON-ON!" (Hasher speak for "Keep running") I heard. It was Jonathan (Faith's husband). "You got it, you own it, you're going to Boston!" I knew I was and nodded.

I rounded the corner and saw the Washington Avenue Monster. I also call it the "Mound of Hurt." It's so bad that the race directors spray paint "I'M SORRY," at the bottom of it. As I hit the bottom of it I saw him at the top. Unmistakably in his blue shorts, blue bandana, and pencil thin legs, it was Dave Kennedy. He had faded. He had about 0.4 miles to go and about 3:30, for a 3:10.59 chip, to do it. It was going to be close. "RUN DAVE! RUNNNNNNNN!" I screamed it with all of the air I had in my lungs.

This caused me to walk the hill a bit about a quarter of the way up.

"Come with me. Baby steps," said the woman who I talked into running about a mile back. I ran along side her and then started picking it up. I came to 26, near the Scranton Cultural Center with an 8:18. My watch said 3:11:11. I was going.

"Great run, Jay! You're home!" shouted committee member Kevin Calpin.

As I came over the top and onto Washington and Mulberry, there were Mom and Aunt Evelyn (the wife of Unk); pinch-hitting in my Dad's spot was my son, Julian. Couldn't find a better person for the job. They were cheering.

"Pack my bags. We're going to Boston!" I shouted to them.

I came down the final chute and Mike and Kristi Kozlansky were cheering me in. "C'mon Jay! Finish strong!" Mike insisted. When Mike insists, you do it. As I was wondering what time he finished to be in the crowd already, I broke into the fastest run I had. There would be nothing left in the tank. Either of them.

[It was then that it happened—"The Shart Heard 'Round the World." In my ecstasy, I sharted myself. I didn't even break stride. I couldn't care less.]

"I'M GOING TO BOSTON! I'M GOING TO BOSTON!"

I had qualified for the Boston Marathon and Downtown Scranton was going to know it. They roared back. These are my people. I am their rock star. (This attitude inspired by and courtesy of ego prostitute Gene Simmons....)

I actually saw my wife in the finishing chute this time. First time in six years. (I think the red jacket helped...) I crossed the line in 3:12.42. Multiplying by 2 and adding 10 was right again. It was the most unreal feeling. I can't describe it, but the picture captures it perfectly. I got into the chute, high fived and hugged my way through the crowd. Kim Stampien (marathoner dentist) clipped off my chip, and Spike Lynott, very fittingly I might add, put the finisher's medal around my neck.

I was in another world. I could have died at that moment and been content.

I eyed Dave Kennedy. He was limping. "Did you make it?" I asked trying to will the answer to be a yes.

He shook his head no. "I missed it by 20 seconds."

From the thrill of victory to the agony of defeat in a microsecond.

I broke down into tears and hugged my friend. I knew how bad he wanted it. I knew how hard he trained and raced. I knew what it felt like to miss by such a small margin. I was devastated.

We parted ways again, and I went over to my family. The party had begun. Ann Williams (great family friend) was snapping pictures and even hugged my sweaty body. Her daughter Melissa was not so apt to do so. My aunt, mom, wife, son, Dave (father-in-law) and family friend Michael Rahl gathered together. We were celebrating and remembering our fallen relatives.

My aunt did not know about my tribute to Unk on my singlet. She saw it and kissed it—on my sweaty back she kissed it. She loved the man and was honored by the tribute.

We all went our separate ways, but would meet up later at my post race party.

"To finish is to win, but to qualify is ecstasy."

Seconds from the finish of my Boston Qualifying 2006 Steamtown

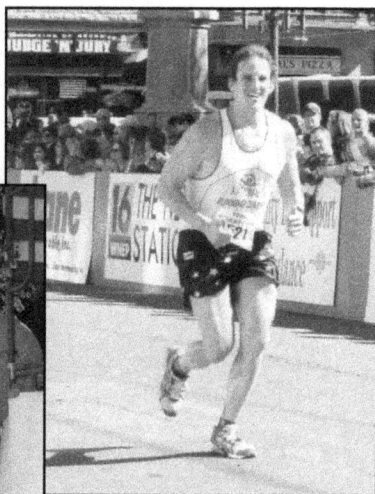

Sheer Ecstacy

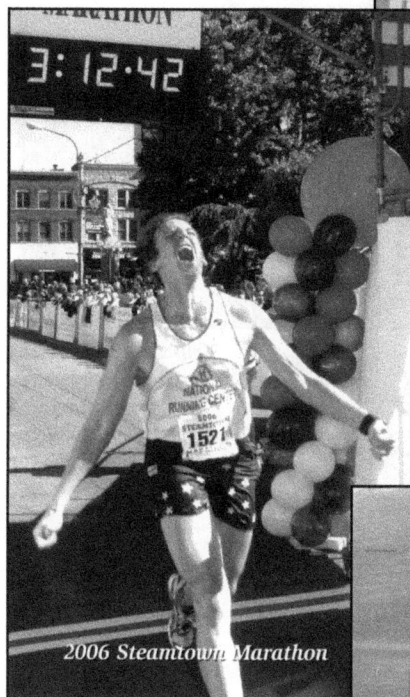

2006 Steamtown Marathon

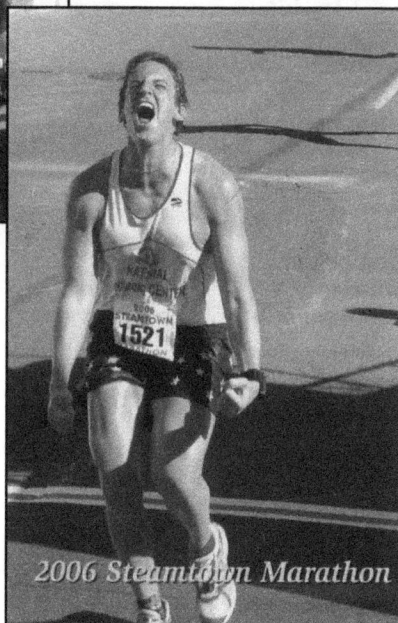

Still in the moment a microsecond later

2006 Steamtown Marathon

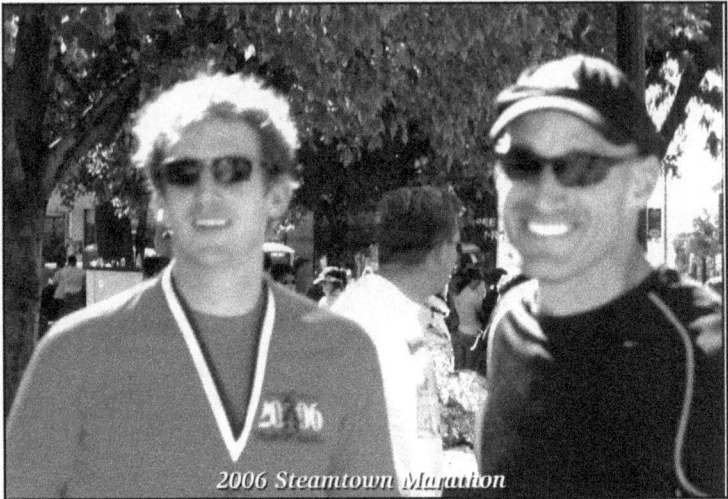

2006 Steamtown Marathon

*Ironman Finisher
Mike Kozlansky and
myself post-race.
He beat me by half a day
or something like that.*

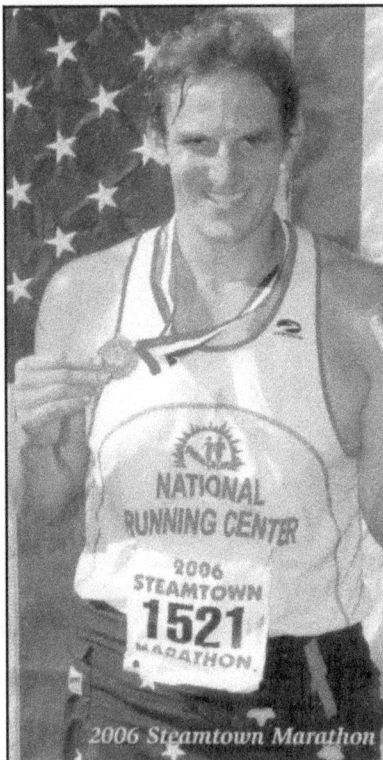

NATIONAL
RUNNING CENTER

2006
STEAMTOWN
1521
MARATHON

2006 Steamtown Marathon

*Post Boston Qualifying
afterglow. Like I said,
I'm a rockstar!*

18

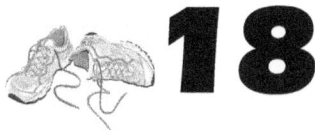

The Boston Saga
Part I

I T is such a cascade in my mind that I barely know where to start.

The day had finally arrived. Saturday, April 14, 2007, 8 a.m. Departure for Boston was imminent. My community of Covington Township was wishing me well since the beginning of April. It felt as if they would be vicariously running the Boston Marathon with me. Even my Chinese food was on my side. The fortune cookie read, "Sometimes travel to new places leads to great transformation."

My son Julian's kindergarten class made me a card that could only be produced by five-year-olds. 'Wine the ras," it said, along with other humorous misspellings. The card lifted my already high spirits, and I looked at it often over race weekend.

The traveling party consisted of Sheryl, Julian, Mom, Aunt Evelyn and my friends, Frank and Beki Kosydar Krantz; their daughter, Corah; and Beki's Aunt Joanne. As we set off, I wanted to get some sleep in the van, but I was too excited. I spent most of the ride talking with Frank, who still holds Lakeland High School pole-vaulting records from the late '80s. Frank was instrumental in helping me develop my focus on race day.

The van pulled into a Perkin's Restaurant and it was time to carboload.

I ordered the ham-and-cheese omelet (protein and necessary fats) with hash browns and pancakes along with an additional short stack of French toast. My inner fat man was ecstatic. Jo Ellen, our server, was an absolute doll. On our check, she wished me good luck in the marathon. I ripped off the bottom of the check and carried it to Boston.

Before we knew it I was at the Best Western, in Revere, Mass. As I entered our room, I saw it out of the corner of my eye: The navy blue 2007 Image Impact Boston Marathon jacket wrapped around the frame of another runner.

"Nice jacket," I said.

"You too," was the reply.

Her name is Terry, and she qualified for her first Boston in 2006 in Philadelphia. She had her husband, Brett, and twin daughters, Kyra and Holly in tow. She was from Emmaus, PA, which made us practically neighbors. We became instant friends.

There was a nor'easter looming on the horizon, and Sheryl felt a migraine coming on. She opted to rest while I checked out the expo. The front desk gave me directions, but it turned out all I had to do was follow the jackets. Boston was being temporarily leased by 20,000 runners. It was our town, and we were determined to take it by storm.

19

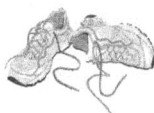

The Boston Saga
Part II

THE expo was smaller than I expected.
I have seen corporate expos twice the size, but runners are more of a niche group. The crowd was small, but the vibe was massive. You could almost see the energy transfer from one runner to another. Tights were fashionable, and the Garmin forerunner was considered a classy watch. I wore my retro Ironman. (My first running watch. Before that, I used the bank clock). I was looking around casually, bought some gels at National Running Center, and then ran into the *Marathon & Beyond* expo booth.

I was looking around the display and noticed a card that read, "Pam Reed." The name instantly clicked. She was the woman who twice won Badwater—a 135-mile race against dehydration and death that starts in 120-degree Death Valley and ends on the top of a mountain.

Pam was also the first runner to run 300 consecutive miles, and she was standing right next to me. I was a bit starstruck, but managed not to gush too much. I think she was just as impressed with my story, at least the weight loss part. Pam signed 5829 (my race bib) and then a man, noticing my camera, asked if I wanted him to take our pic-

ture. It was a video camera, so I interviewed her. Rich Be-
nyo (*M&B*'s editor) asked if I did that for a living. I don't. I
just don't mind the camera being there. I then did the same
thing with Rich.

I meandered around again and signed the Promise Wall
and Book. I then filled out an Adidas bib for why I run. I
promised to give it all I had for 26.2 and to run for Dad and
Uncle Mike. I always do. On the bib I wrote that I ran to
show the world what a former 300-pounder could do in a
marathon. I immersed myself in the whole experience.

Then I saw her in front of the Runner's World display.
#261. Kathy Switzer. The first registered woman to run
Boston.

I immediately bought her autobiography, which she
signed, and had her autograph my race bib as well. She
signs it upside down so you can see it while you race. We
kind of interviewed each other. She was asking me questions about my first Boston. I asked her about her famous
encounter with Jock Semple who tried to grab her and pull
her off the course.

I woke up Sunday morning very well rested. I knew that
I would not get a lot of sack time the night before the race.
I was already excited. I decided to take my traditional two-
mile hop before we went to Church (also a pre-race ritual).
It was cloudy and starting to rain. I was in shorts and a
light thermal shirt to test the weather a bit. I was cold for
the first half-mile then I broke a pretty good sweat. By the
time I got back to the hotel, it was raining sideways.

Instantly, I was glad that this was not a Sunday race. I
got changed, hopped a cab and went to church. St. Anthony's is an old-school place of worship. The Mass was great.
The organist was absolutely phenomenal. I stayed around

for his last note just so I could clap for him. It was practically a concert.

As we waited for a cab, an old man asked if I would walk him to his car. He had horrible neurological impairment. It looked like advanced Parkinson's Disease to me. Thoughts of my Dad immediately flooded my mind. I'm glad it was raining so no one saw me cry as I walked him to his car. It was very emotional. In a way I was glad. It felt like I got to touch a piece of Dad that day. It was his way of saying "Hello" as I got ready for the race. Our cab arrived, we went to the hotel and got ready for an excursion to Boston.

We got on the T and set out for the Boston Aquarium, which was packed with runners watching the potential disaster set up outside. You could feel the tension. I swear that every runner I talked to was from San Diego, and "The weather was never like this." We finished up and headed to the aquarium. The short walk was miserable — thousands of blue and white jackets looking ruefully up at the angry sky.

There were rumors that the race would be canceled, but I don't think that was ever an option. People plan this trip months, often years, in advance. The logistics of such a race are mind boggling. You can't just have a rain date the next week. By evening, the rain was accompanied by gale-force winds blowing in from the sea. This meant a headwind for the race, and I think it was around midnight before I nodded off to the sound of wind and rain slamming against the window.

The 4 a.m. wake-up call came around fast. We had to be on the buses by 6:30. I went down to the lobby to grab some breakfast and, you guessed it, ran into Terry. We ate and talked a bit. We were both hyped up.

"I can't believe I'll be running with the world's best today," I said.

"Take a look at your bib number," she said. "You're one of them."

Wow! I thought to myself.

She had a point. Number 5829 out of 23,000. I was up there a bit. We said goodbye and I hopped the airport shuttle Hopkinton High School and the start of the race.

I was dressed for a battle with the elements. I opted to wear a top under my singlet, banking on a steady rain to keep me from overheating. I also packed latex gloves for my hands. Two or three pairs will keep you warm as toast. You can also peel them to adjust your comfort level.

The first mile reminded me of Route 171 around miles two through six in the Steamtown Marathon: Houses and trees all around with the hill doing the work for you. Everyone was in front of their houses or on their porches. I heard people playing music and cheering for all 20,000 of us. It was once again the rock star treatment. We were the heroes of the day.

I was also starting to feel the effects of going out at that fast a pace. I really didn't kill myself training for Boston. Winter got to me this year and it cut into the amount of 20-milers that I put in. Within three miles I was already running 7:40's. I simply did not have the legs to sustain anything near my Steamtown pace.

I wasn't kidding myself. I knew a PR was not in my immediate future. I had made a decision.

Jonathan Loiselle came up from behind me. I told him that "I just didn't have it today." I decided to make this a 26-mile celebration of my accomplishments. I went into pleasure cruise mode and had fun with it. Since I was going to have fun, I decided to make myself comfortable. I hit the first port-o-john I saw. I took off my two shirts, took care of business, and got back on the course.

I was chilly for about 30 seconds; then I was fine. I also removed my bandanna and gloves a little later. Staying warm was not a problem. I had to get rid of my shirt. By this time I was in Ashland and there was a nice crowd in the town. I pulled a "Mean Joe Green" and tossed my shirt to a kid. I couldn't tell if she was awed by the gesture or mortified to be holding the sweaty thing. I'm thinking the latter.

After this, something amazing happened. I never heard him come up on me, and I lost sight of him in a blink, but I'll never forget what he said.

"Your Dad is damn proud of you right now."

I said, "Thanks, man," and he was gone. I am an un-abashedly spiritual person. I totally believe that I was de-livered a personal message. Sure, the speaker could have seen the "DAD 1-22-05" on my shirt, but he didn't have to say a thing about it. Once again, Dad somehow managed to say how proud he was of my running. I will never forget the moment.

I high-fived my way from town to town. People were cheering for "Mr. USA", "Captain America", and doing the "U-S-A" cheer. It kept me going. So did the downhill. I was told that it was downhill to 16, up for four, then downhill.

So far, they were right. I had 20 and "Heartbreak Hill" on my mind. I heard from the Scranton bunch that it was really overrated and that "People there don't know what hills are." I had a way to go, but the thought was there. I did not need a knock-down-drag-out hill set like Steamtown.

At 12.5 I heard it: "The Scream." A half-mile out and you could hear the Wellesley girls.

Runners were disappointed. Usually it's a mile out. I felt like the Sixth Beatle (never forget Pete Best). That is the only sound I could compare it to—either the Beatles in 1964 or the screams on Cheap Trick's "Live at Budokan." There were signs that said "Kiss me." I obliged the request. Felt it was my duty.

One of the "Kiss me" signs belonged to a guy. I figured he was aiming at a different demographic, but I stopped, grabbed him by the back of the head and planted one on his cheek. I stuck it there, too. The release produced an audible "smack." The girls around him were in hysterics.

I had the time of my life and floated from town to town. With the exception of Wellesley, I couldn't tell you the order of them or where they are on the course. It was just one continuous runner fan club. I heard cheers for Holland, London, Korea and the name of everyone who had a name on their shirt. It was totally uplifting.

At 16, the hills started. At worst, they were rollers in the beginning. There was plenty of time to recover from one to the other. The general grade was gently uphill at most. I was having no problem climbing my way up the course.

The overdressed fared far worse. There were people wearing the official Blue-and-White jacket while running the race. The sweat was absolutely pouring off of them. I felt bad about tossing a $30 shirt.

I heard the story of a runner who gave his jacket to a fan along with his address so he would mail it home for him. Not a bad idea, but that's what throwaways are for. No matter where you are from, temps in the 40s equal shorts weather for a runner. Within a few miles, you sweat. (They donate tossed clothes to a shelter, so don't feel bad about throwing them away.)

For years, the Hash House Harriers have had a beer stop at the base of Heartbreak Hill. I took my gulp of liquid courage (Sam Adams) and hit it hard. I was on the beast. It was just the two of us. I looked up and already saw the top. "That's it?" I said to myself.

I felt like Peppermint Patty in *A Charlie Brown Thanksgiving*. I was expecting turkey and I got toast with popcorn.

"You did it! You're up Heartbreak Hill!" cheered a bunch.

"THAT WAS IT?! THAT WAS NOTHING! COME TO SCRANTON, AND I'LL SHOW YOU SOME HILLS!" I shouted. Yes, I talked some smack to the Heartbreak faithful. Much like the Super Bowl, the hype was greater than the event. Steamtown's hills are much tougher.

"It's all downhill from here!" the crowd cheered.

I was totally in the zone, living off the energy of the crowd. I was so focused on them that I ran past Fenway Park without seeing it; big green thing on the right with a lot of people wearing Red Sox hats. Ran right by it. Never saw it.

I took the last looping turn, went a block and made a left onto Boyleston Street. With sore arms I high-fived my way down the left-hand side. I took it all in as I crossed the finish line and celebrated all of my accomplishments. I lived in every moment of that race. I was thrilled to be a part of it.

Still, I was disappointed with my effort. About 1 percent of me was appalled by my time. 6,900 out of 20,000 in 3:35ish is not bad for celebrating and killing a lot of time. The fact is that I did not have many other options. The greatest race in the world, and I didn't give it my best race. I couldn't. It wasn't there to give. It will never happen again.

We came home to a foot of snow. Not the homecoming I expected. The party was over. Time to return to the hum-drum of everyday life after three glorious days as a running rock star. It was all downhill from Boston, but when you've got the support of a loving family and the drive to find and con-quer the next hill, you learn to appreciate a well-earned lull.

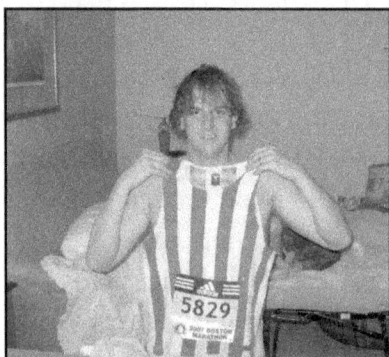

4 a.m. race morning

Post-race with the Mrs.

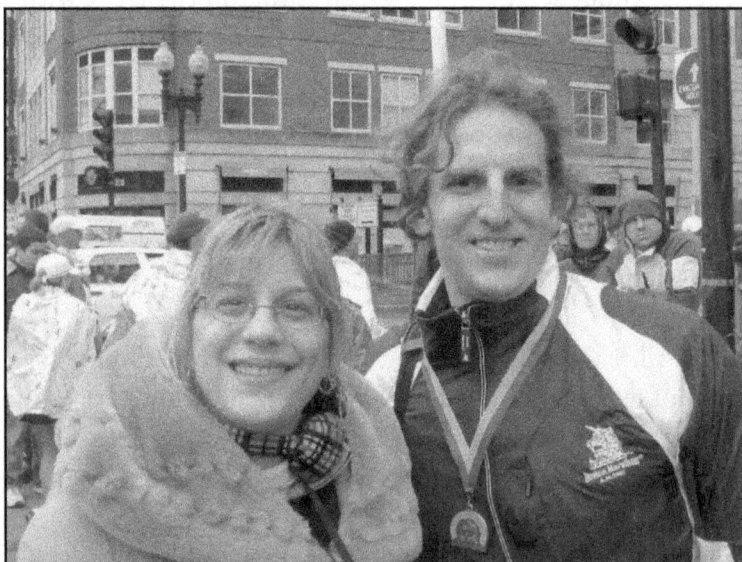

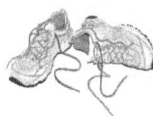

20

Epilogue

As of this writing, it has been three years since I ran Boston. The achievement of that goal is something I could not have begun to imagine 10 years ago. I truly have been blessed. That is not to say that what I have done was just handed to me. There was a lot of hard work involved from starting as the Red Headed Fat Kid and winding up a Boston Marathon finisher. It may not have been easy, but it was totally worth it.

I may have busted his chops in a line or two of this book, but Gene Simmons is a hero of mine. He came to America as an Israeli immigrant with absolutely nothing and wound up an entertainment mogul with wealth beyond imagination. I remember reading an interview of his in *Metal Edge* magazine. He succinctly described the secret to his success. To paraphrase him (I'm too lazy to research the exact quote), he said that you can be successful at anything as long as you are willing to put in the hard work it takes to get there. I believe he is right.

I put in thousands of miles of running to run the Boston Marathon. I got up many times before the sun in the freezing cold to get my runs in. I also sacrificed time away from my family so I could train.

I had a lot of work to do just to get to the point of being able to run ¼ mile. I had to lose over 100 pounds. I had to develop a new set of rules for living my life. I had to learn portion control and work exercise into my routine. I never say that "I went on a diet" to describe how I lost the weight and kept it off. I say that I underwent a lifestyle renovation.

Losing the weight is relatively easy compared to keeping it off. For ten years now, it has been a constant battle. It always seems like there is a holiday or another event that I have to contend with in my schedule. In Weight Watchers, there is a term called "maintenance." Once you have lost the weight, you play around with your *POINTS* until you find the magic number when you are not losing and not gaining weight. I have no idea what that number is for me. It seems like I am always recovering from a holiday and I have been trying to lose 10 more pounds for I have no idea how long now. I'll tell you this. I'd rather be trying to lose the same 10 pounds than the same 100 again. I may battle my weight for the rest of my life but it's a fight I'm willing to take on.

If you are heavy and want to lose weight, remember that I have been where you have been. I've told myself that I was happy with myself when I was actually miserable being fat. I used the line, "If God wanted me thin, He would have made me that way." I knew that wasn't true either. I felt absolutely powerless to do anything with my weight and that my life had become unmanageable. I felt like I had lost the war.

When I took my stand and said "enough is enough," I was standing on the cliff of my life. I was 306 pounds. One of two things was going to happen. I was going to go up to 400, or even 500, pounds or I was going to go down to 200. There is no doubt in my mind that it could have gone the other way. I am thankful to God that it didn't.

In dieting terms, I am an asterisk. I am the asterisk at the bottom of your TV screen or magazine add that says "*Results not typical." I say that it is time for the asterisk to become the norm. It is time for this country to say "Enough!" This country is standing on a precipice. Usually, the next generation outlives the previous one. That's the way it has been since the dawn of time. Advances of healthcare have extended human life to the point where dying at age 70 is considered young. Human behavior may override medical science. Some people are predicting that my child's generation will not outlive mine. I believe they may be correct. We need to change that. We need to save our children.

I have seen it in my profession. When I first was a pharmacy intern, it seemed like people were fine into their mid-forties, then they needed medication for blood pressure, high cholesterol, or diabetes. My, how times have changed. This now starts with people in their early thirties, and I have even seen people as young as 20 on such medications. Frankly, I think the medications are to blame. They make it easy to manage the conditions. Why go on a diet and exercise when you can make it all better by taking a pill?

The answer to that is simple. The medication is like putting a Band-Aid on the Hoover Dam to stop a leak. It's not going to hold. Eventually, the disease is going to win. Eventually, you are going to have a heart attack or stroke out. Eventually, due to your high cholesterol, you are going to clog a coronary artery. Due to your out of control glucose levels, you are going to develop leg ulcers, ruin your kidneys, or even lose your vision. That can all be simply avoided.

The first-line (and greatly overlooked) defense in all three of the above mentioned diseases is lifestyle modification (diet, exercise, and smoking cessation). Unless you are genetically predisposed to such conditions, taking those three steps can save your life without ever having to pop a pill.

Believe me when I tell you that you can do this. You can change your life and get down to a healthy weight. How do I know this? I did it; that's how I know. I'm not special. I don't possess any super power that makes me stronger than the human race. I am just a flawed human being. I am no different that you. I did it and so can you.

Since you know that you can do it, I guess you are wondering, "'How can I do this?" You'll have to buy my next book *How I Did It* by Jay Sochoka, R.Ph. to find out. (Just kidding.)

As a health care professional (pharmacists do a lot more than just count to 30), and as someone who did it, here is what I suggest.

1) Go to Weight Watchers. Forget Atkins, forget Jenny Craig, and forget NutriSystem. Weight Watchers teaches you how to live. It just makes sense. You will learn portion control and how to care for yourself. You won't just eat pre-packaged foods; you will learn how to cook healthy. You will develop habits that you will take with you for the rest of your life.

2) Weigh, measure, and write down everything that goes into your mouth. Once you learn portion control, life in the lifestyle modification world gets a lot easier. Do NOT "eyeball" measurements. You will almost certainly underestimate how much something actually is.

3) Find an exercise that you like and stick with it. Walking, running, cycling, and swimming are four that quickly come to mind. There are literally thousands of gyms, exercise books, videos, and pieces of home equipment out

there. There has to be something you can incorporate into your life from all that is out there. Remember all you need to start walking is a good pair of sneakers. Everything else you already own. You can get started for cheap.

4) Hydrate. Drink 6-8 eight ounce glasses of water everyday. It helps you body run more efficiently and, when imbibed with your meals, helps you feel fuller longer. It's a trick that I have been using for a long time and it works.

5) Get five servings of fruits and vegetables everyday. I hate to sound like one of the pundits, but when they're right, they're right. It's important to diversify in your diet and fruits and veggies are a good way to do it. The fiber will help you feel full and a high fiber diet has been proven to reduce your cholesterol.

6) Don't deprive yourself. That directly leads to failure. I'm not saying to treat yourself everyday, but, once in a while, live a little. If you're doing Weight Watchers, you can even "legally" do this. Every food has a *POINTS* value. If you are willing to spend the *POINTS*, you can eat anything you want while on Weight Watchers. The question is "Are you willing to blow all of your *POINTS* on it everyday?" I hope the answer is "no," because you won't feel full and will probably backslide. Remember that everything in life is fair game as long as it is done in moderation. Moderation, however, can be a tricky state to maintain. The bottom line is to treat yourself but do it only on occasion.

7) Be patient with yourself when starting a new lifestyle program. You didn't gain all of the weight in one day, one month, or most likely one year. It took years for you to get where you are. It may take years for you to get to where you want to be. You are not going to see six-pack abs after one week of crunches (how I wish that wasn't true), so please

be patient. You are going to get to that goal weight, but remember that this process is a marathon and not a sprint.

I talk about the Inner Fatman a lot in this book, and here is what I mean. It does not matter what I look like, I know that I can take in a ridiculous amount of food. I could out eat Michael Phelps during the Olympics.

I don't like to eat, I love to binge. I don't like feeling satisfied, I love feeling gorged! The only reason I know that I have eaten enough food is because my food journal told me that I have done so. My favorite holiday is Thanksgiving, because it pays tribute to my two favorite deadly sins. Sloth and gluttony. This is who my Inner Fatman is.

Every so often, I like to give my Inner Fatman a great, big, can't get my arms around him, hug. I like to do this on holidays. Like I said Thanksgiving is my #1 fave, but I like to celebrate all that are on the calendar. I said I celebrate them. I'm not going to eat a salad while everyone else is eating a rack of ribs. I'm going to enjoy the holiday. I'm not going to make it a holiweek, holimonth, or holiyear.

The very next day I'm going to get my food journal out and get back on the horse. You WILL fall off the horse once in a while. We all do. Success is measured in how quickly you could jump up, dust off, and get back in the saddle after you are thrown off.

In the last installment of the *Rocky* series, the main character said this. "It's not how hard you're hit. It's how hard you can get hit, how much you can take, and keep moving forward. That's how winning is done!"

You may be saying, "OK. I'll give it a try." I will quote Master Yoda in *The Empire Strikes Back* and say. "No! Try not. Do or do not. There is no try." This has been a mantra of mine throughout life. I hope you make it part of yours.

Like I said, I am not perfect. I am horribly flawed. There are days when I don't exercise or track my food. If I see you having a cigarette, chances are that I'll bum one off of you. Okay, maybe two. It is all part of the human condition though. Once you realize that you are not perfect and all knowing, you are ready to succeed. In your weakness, there is strength.

I don't run like I once did. I used to obsess over every mile. I even over-trained to the point of injury once or twice. I used to run to live. It meant everything to me. That feeling is long gone. It has been medicated out of me.

You see, God is not without a sense of irony. I understand my Dad more now than I ever could have in the past. In August of 2005, I was diagnosed with bipolar disorder.

Remember when, two months after my Dad died, I didn't sleep, was laughing one minute then crying the next? That was my first manic episode. I'm doing much better today, but the years in between have not been without their incidents. I did learn this: Dad was a good man with an ugly disease. He did the best he could with what he had and, compared to his father, he came light years.

It is my goal to get further away from the demons than my Dad did. I want to show my son that, should he ever be diagnosed, life does go on and, when properly controlled, bipolar disorder is a beautiful thing. I give credit for my creativity and the writing of this book to the disorder. It makes me who I am, and I wouldn't change that for anything.

I actually skipped the 2008 and 2009 Steamtown Marathons. I had neither the desire nor the need to train for them. And that's okay. I am not defined by whether I run or not anymore. I am a faithful servant, a husband, a father, and a good friend. Running doesn't come close to making that list. It doesn't need to. Will I ever run another marathon? I guarantee you that I will.

I need you to know this. Inside you have your own set of powers, which you have not even begun to tap. With these powers, you will find your inner drive. One you tap into that, you can accomplish anything. Find that power and the sky's the limit.

I fully realize that I have just contradicted myself. Before, I said, "Through Him all things are possible." Now I'm talking about your inner power. So which one is it, you ask?

Both.

God has given us everything we need to do something really spectacular. He puts everything in line for us to do something with it. He gives you this huge pile of wood, but you have to light the match to get the fire burning. He gives you the library, but you have to read the books. He puts you well-trained on the starting line, but you have to run the marathon. I think you get the point.

Speaking of the marathon, treat life like one. Run it easy; don't sprint. Keep a nice steady pace. Remember, for every hill you have to labor to climb, there is one to cruise down in an easy gait. Don't worry about how long it takes you to finish. Just finish. Celebrate the pure victory of success.

People call me thin, and I can't stand it. I have a totally distorted self body image, and I have never seen myself as thin. I have not won the battle of the bulge. The day I say that is the day I put all of the weight back on. I have to fight every day to stay in the shape I'm in. As I have said, it's a fight I am willing to take on every day.

Still, I will never be thin. The best I can be is a Fatman in Recovery.

Shalom!

For bulk orders or more information, please contact
Avventura Press
at 570-876-5817 or email
lee@avventurapress.com

Become a Facebook fan:
Jay Sochoka: Fatman In Recovery

Email Jay at jay@avventurapress.com

www.ingramcontent.com/pod-product-compliance
Lightning Source LLC
La Vergne TN
LVHW011232080426
835509LV00005B/461